THYROID DISORDERS

*A Practical Guide
to Understanding
the Causes and Treatments*

Dr Rowan Hillson

Illustrated by
Maggie Raynor

Vermilion
LONDON

For my grandparents

9 10

First published by Vermilion, an imprint of Ebury Publishing, in 1997
This revised edition published by Vermilion in 2002
First published in the UK in 1991 by Macdonald Optima

Ebury Publishing is a Random House Group company

The Random House Group Limited Reg. No. 954009

Addresses for companies within the Random House Group can be found at
www.randomhouse.co.uk

A CIP catalogue record for this book is available from the British Library

ISBN 9780091884345

Copies are available at special rates for bulk orders. Contact the sales development team on 020 7840 8487 or visit www.booksforpromotions.co.uk for more information.

To buy books by your favourite authors and register for offers, visit
www.randomhouse.co.uk

Penguin Random House is committed to a sustainable future for our business, our readers and our planet. This book is made from Forest Stewardship Council® certified paper.

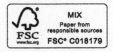

Printed and bound in Great Britain by Clays Ltd, St Ives plc

Contents

Acknowledgements

I thank all the people with thyroid conditions who have shared their experience with me, and the physicians who kindled and maintained my interest in endocrinology. Without these patients and these professionals this book would not have been written.

I am also grateful to the following who contributed to the making and refining of this book: Kate Adams, Jayne Booth, Michael Colston, Harriet Griffey, Kay and Rodney Hillson, Simon Hillson, Mark Lee, Dai Thomas.

1
Introduction

Thyroid disorders are common, particularly in women, but they can be treated. But many more people have abnormalities of thyroid function without realising it, some of whom will come to need treatment.

This book is for people who have thyroid problems, whether overactivity or underactivity; for those who have been told they have minor thyroid abnormalities and for the families of people with thyroid disorders. Nurses and others who work with people who have thyroid trouble may also find it helpful.

The book is written in several sections: the first introduces the thyroid gland and how it works; the second considers the underactive thyroid gland and the third the overactive thyroid gland; the following sections discuss pregnancy, thyroid eye disorders and goitres; then there is a section discussing other conditions which are more likely to occur in people with thyroid disorders than in those without; finally there is a section about looking after yourself and keeping fit. Throughout I have presented the problems from the perspective of the people who have them, starting with what they may notice wrong, followed by the visit to the doctor, diagnosis and treatment. Then I discuss the complications of the conditions and finally their causes.

I have used stories about people with thyroid disorders as examples. None of these people exist though – the names are all fictitious. But the stories do combine observations of many patients I have seen over the years.

One of the difficulties in writing information books for people with medical problems is that there are many ways of assessing, investigating and treating the condition; every doctor has his or her own way of managing the condition. Thyroid disorders are no different – there are many views on all aspects of the conditions. The fact that one doctor advises a different treatment from another does not necessarily mean that one is right and one is wrong – there are several ways of managing the same conditions, all of which are accepted and successful. I have tried to give an overview of the conditions and their management and an insight into some of the areas of controversy. But it is very important to remember that every person has his or her own unique version of the condition which needs individual attention from his or her doctor.

One of the aims of this book is to encourage you to think about your own condition and to ask yourself questions about what is happening in your body. Please turn to your doctor to help you answer such questions. He or she is the only one who knows all the details of your own very special case. It is also extremely important that you do not change your treatment without first discussing it with your doctor.

In Britain, it is usually your general practitioner who will diagnose your thyroid disorder, although – as you will see in this book – thyroid problems have many disguises and can take you to a variety of specialist clinics before being recognised. Many general practitioners are happy to manage patients with thyroid insufficiency, although should refer all those who are pregnant or under 16 years of age to a specialist. All patients with newly diagnosed thyroid over-activity should have the opportunity of seeing a specialist. Doctors specialising in the management of hormone disorders are called endocrinologists. Diabetes is usually considered as a separate, though linked, hormone speciality. In most instances, the majority of an endocrinologist's patients will have thyroid disorders. The endocrinologist will then liaise with your general practitioner about your care.

In this book, I have referred to your doctor as 'he' for convenience, although as a woman doctor I am well aware that many doctors are female! No offence is intended.

Over the years you may move around the country or travel abroad. Remember that once you have been diagnosed as having a thyroid problem, you should have your thyroid status checked at least once a year for ever, no matter where you are.

I believe that people should know the proper names for parts of their body, and that those who are unwell should know the medical terms for their condition and the tests and treatments relating to it. I have therefore used these terms throughout the book, but always with explanations. There is also a glossary at the end which explains most of the medical and scientific words used in this book (see pages 171–180).

2

The Thyroid Gland

The thyroid gland lies in the neck. It is divided into two parts, a right and a left lobe, resting on either side of the Adam's apple. These lobes are linked by a narrow band of tissue called the isthmus. The thyroid gland is partly covered by the strap-like sternomastoid muscles that run from just below the angle of the jaw to the knobbles of the collarbones

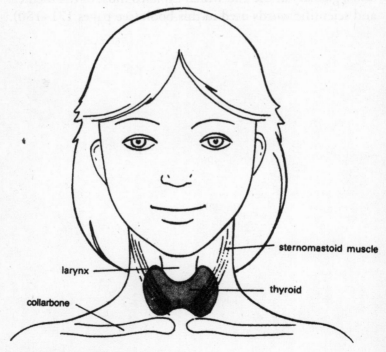

The thyroid gland in the neck.

where they join the breastbone. You may be able to feel your thyroid – slip your fingers gently under the sternomastoid muscle and run them down on either side of the Adam's apple and the trachea (the windpipe); the thyroid is a softish tissue which goes up and down on swallowing.

In the unborn baby the thyroid gland starts life as a small piece of tissue at the back of the tongue and gradually migrates down the neck to its adult site.

Thyroid Hormones

Like most body tissues the thyroid gland has a good blood supply, providing it with nutrients and removing waste substances. Because it is a gland, i.e. it produces secretions, these blood vessels also carry away the chemicals – the secretions – that the thyroid produces. These chemicals then travel in the bloodstream to all the parts of the body where they exert their effect. Such chemical messengers, produced by a small gland but acting throughout the body, are called hormones, and the glands that produce them – in this case the thyroid – are called endocrine glands. The hormones made by the thyroid are called thyroxine (T4 for short) and tri-iodothyronine (T3 for short).

If you look at the thyroid under a microscope you can see that it is made up of round balls of functioning tissue, called follicles. The follicles are set in non-functioning connective tissue through which the blood vessels run. Each follicle consists of a wall of follicular cells enclosing a gel-like centre called colloid. The follicular cells are the tiny factories which make thyroid hormones, and the colloid acts as a storage depot for thyroid hormones.

The raw materials for thyroid hormone manufacture are carried to the follicular cells by the bloodstream, the main raw material being iodine. We need about 100 to 200 micrograms of iodine a day, which we obtain from the food we eat. The iodine is transferred into the follicular cell from the bloodstream and chemically processed into thyroid hormone precursors – the chemicals from which thyroid hormones are made. At the same time, the follicular cell makes a special carrier substance called thyroglobulin. The iodine-containing hormone precursors are bound to the thyroglobulin, which oozes out of the follicular cell into the colloid. There the precursors undergo further chemical processing to produce T3 (which contains three iodine units) and T4 (which contains four iodine units). The mixtures of T3/T4/thyroglobulin are then stored in the colloid in the centre of the follicle. When the thyroid hormones are needed the follicular cells take in tiny globules

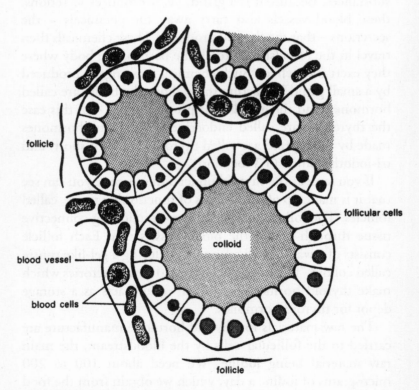

Thyroid follicles as seen under a microscope.

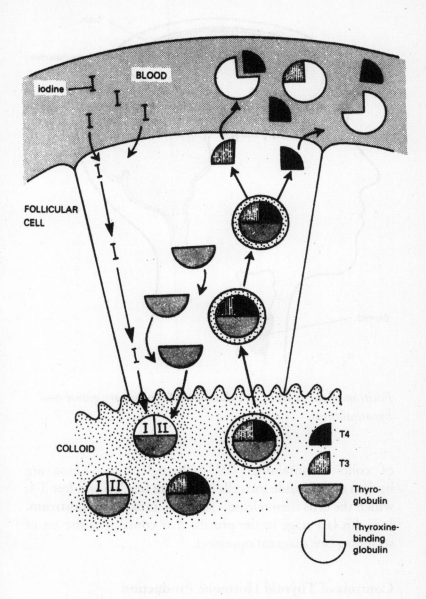

How thyroid hormone is manufactured in the follicular cell and released into the bloodstream.

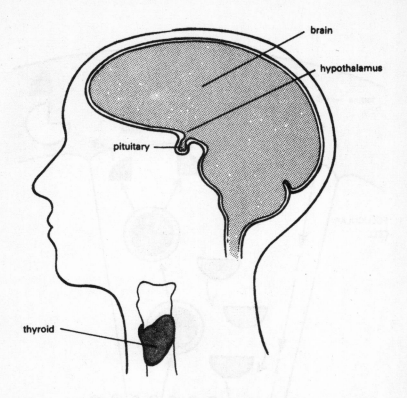

Position of the thyroid in relation to the pituitary gland and hypothalamus.

of colloid containing T3/T4/thyroglobulin. These are broken down inside the cells to liberate free T3 and free T4, which the cells then release – secrete – into the bloodstream. It is this last stage in the process that constitutes the act of secretion (see diagram opposite).

Controls of Thyroid Hormone Production

The thyroid gland is thus rather like a factory. Throughout the day the bloodstream delivers iodine and other raw materials, and the thyroid makes them into T4 and T3 to be delivered to the rest of the body. But the thyroid gland itself has no control over the amount of T4 and T3 it makes; that is decided by the factory's head office – the pituitary gland, another endocrine gland.

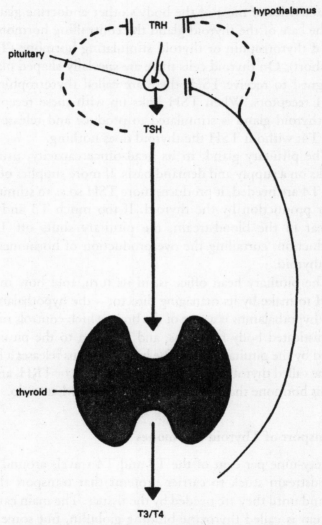

The relationship between the hypothalamus, pituitary and thyroid in the production of thyroid hormone.

The pituitary gland lies in a tiny bony chamber in the base of the skull. It is no bigger than a thumbnail in diameter, but is one of the most powerful organs in the body. Linked to the brain by a narrow stalk of tissue, the pituitary gland produces its own hormones which control the activities of most of the body's other endocrine glands. In the case of the thyroid gland the controlling hormone is called thyrotrophin or thyroid stimulating hormone (TSH for short). On thyroid cells there are specially-shaped places designed to receive TSH; these are called thyrotrophin or TSH receptors. When TSH links up with these receptors the thyroid gland is stimulated to produce and release T3 and T4: without TSH the thyroid does nothing.

The pituitary gland, in its head-office capacity, usually works on a supply and demand basis. If more supplies of T3 and T4 are needed, it produces more TSH so as to stimulate their production by the thyroid. If too much T3 and T4 appear in the bloodstream, the pituitary shuts off TSH production, curtailing the overproduction of hormones by the thyroid.

The pituitary head office is, in its turn, told how much TSH to make by its managing director – the hypothalamus. The hypothalamus is a part of the brain which controls many sophisticated body functions, and is linked to the pituitary gland by the pituitary stalk. The hypothalamus releases a hormone called thyrotrophin-releasing hormone, or TRH, and it is this hormone that tells the pituitary gland what to do.

Transport of Thyroid Hormones

Ninety-nine per cent of the T3 and T4 travels around the bloodstream stuck to carrier proteins that transport them around until they are needed by the tissues. The main carrier protein is called thyroxine-binding globulin, but some T3 and T4 is also bound to a protein called albumin, and the rest is free in the blood.

With older methods of thyroid-hormone measurement this linkage with carrier proteins in the blood can sometimes lead to confusion; for instance, if there is a high blood protein level (such as can occur in women taking a contraceptive pill, for example), there can appear to be a high blood total T3 and total T4 level. Newer methods of analysis have resolved this problem by measuring free T3 and free T4 concentrations, so that the answer is not affected by blood protein level. There are about 9–23 picomols of free T4 per litre of blood and 3.5–6.5 picomols of free T3 per litre of blood, although each laboratory may quote slightly different normal ranges depending on their assay methods (methods of analysis) and other local factors. (A picomol is an extremely small unit of concentration, i.e. T3 and T4 are present in the bloodstream in very low concentrations.)

When the thyroid hormones reach the tissues which need them they separate from the carrier proteins and pass into the cells. T4 is not chemically active, however, and has to be converted to T3 before it can be used by the body. This conversion occurs in the liver, kidney, brain and other tissues, including the pituitary gland. In contrast the T3 made by the thyroid gland can be used straightaway.

What Do Thyroid Hormones Do?

Thyroid hormones influence all the major body systems. T3 acts mainly within the cell nucleus (the central core of the cell) where it links to special receptors. Thyroid hormones also exert powerful effects on the tiny parts of cells called mitochondria, in which many essential chemical processes occur, and are needed for other chemical reactions. They influence the mechanisms by which fluids and chemicals enter and leave the cells.

In practical terms the effects of the thyroid hormones can best be seen by noting what goes wrong when a person makes too many or too few. This will be discussed in detail in subsequent chapters, but in general, the right amounts of thyroid hormones are essential for:

- Mental composure and alertness.
- Growth.
- Blood fat balance.
- Strong and steady heart function and blood circulation.
- Balancing the appetite, bowel function and body weight.
- Fluid balance in the body.
- Muscle strength.
- Ability to fight infections.

Summary

- The thyroid gland is in the neck.
- It makes the thyroid hormones tri-iodothyronine, or T3, and thyroxine, or T4.
- The thyroid hormones are made in follicles by the follicular cells and stored in the colloid of the follicles.
- Iodine is the main raw material for thyroid hormone manufacture.
- Thyroid hormone production is controlled by thyroid stimulating hormone, or TSH, which is produced by the pituitary gland in the head. TSH production is in turn controlled by the hypothalamus in the brain.
- T3 and T4 travel around the bloodstream linked with proteins.
- T4 is inactive and is converted to T3 for use by the tissues.
- Thyroid hormones influence all major body systems, the right amounts being essential for normal body functioning.

3
Underactive Thyroid – Symptoms

There are two words to describe an underactive thyroid – hypothyroidism (*hypo* means low) and myxoedema (spelt myxedema in America). Myxoedema was named by William Ord in 1878, although states now known to be due to thyroid insufficiency had been described earlier. Myxoedema (*myx* means mucus, while *oedema* means swelling) strictly speaking describes the firm non-watery swelling that sometimes occurs in the skin of people who have had untreated hypothyroidism for a long time; the term should be applied only to people with this problem, but long usage has made it more generally applicable. For this reason I will use it from now on in this book, simply because I want to avoid any confusion between the words hypothyroidism (underactive thyroid) and hyperthyroidism (overactive thyroid) – two words that look very similar on paper, but which are so very different in people.

Symptoms of an Underactive Thyroid

A symptom is something you notice yourself. This chapter therefore considers the changes and feelings you may have noticed in yourself, one or more of which may have led you to seek medical help, if you have had an underactive thyroid. I have described the symptoms grouped together under the body system affected. This means that common and rare symptoms are listed together. The accompanying table will show you which symptoms are most frequently experienced. Remember that in most people thyroid underactivity is detected early enough to prevent severe symptoms developing. Furthermore, no one person should expect to have all these symptoms. The symptoms of myxoedema are temporary and they usually get better with thyroid hormone replacement treatment.

How common are the symptoms of myxoedema?

Symptom	Percentage of people with myxoedema who have the symptom
Weakness	99
Dry skin	97
Coarse skin	97
Lethargy	91
Slow speech	91
Swollen eyelids	90
Feeling cold	89
Decreased sweating	89
Cold skin	83
Thick tongue	82
Swollen face	79
Coarse hair	76
Pale skin	67
Forgetfulness	66
Constipation	61
Weight gain	59
Hair loss	57
Pale lips	57
Shortness of breath	55
Swollen hands/feet	55
Hoarse voice	52
Loss of appetite	45

Nervousness	35
Heavy periods	32
Palpitations	31
Deafness	30
Chest pain	25

General Appearance

Dry skin, dry hair and brittle nails The skin gradually loses its oils and starts to flake. Women may notice this before men; for example, you may find that you need more moisturiser on your face. Your hands become dry and the skin becomes rather dull and lacklustre. The dry skin may be itchy, and you may notice thickened pads over the knees and elbows. You may not sweat as much as usual, which in turn contributes to your dry skin. Your hair also becomes dull, coarse and dry, and may start to fall out, so that some people who have had unrecognized myxoedema for a long time can develop very thin hair. Furthermore the hair becomes brittle and harder to control. Hair also grows more slowly than usual, and therefore you may find that you need to shave less often and visit the hairdresser or barber less frequently. Your eyebrows may thin out as well. Your nails may become pale or white, grow slowly and break easily. They may develop ridges.

Sallow complexion You may develop a sallow complexion – the skin colour becomes paler and slightly yellowish in general, but the cheeks may become obviously pink or even red. This 'strawberries and cream' complexion is supposedly classical of myxoedema. The yellowness is due to a combination of anaemia and excess carotene in the blood (carotene is an orange-coloured precursor of vitamin A, and myxoedema interferes with its processing in the body). The change in complexion and the very dry skin may lead your beautician to suggest a visit to your doctor. With myxoedema, even if you have a normal blood count your skin may look pale. However, it is not uncommon for people with myxoedema to become anaemic as well, which can make you look very pale. The anaemia is rarely severe, though.

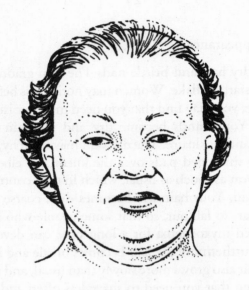

A person with severe myxoedema.

Puffiness, swelling and weight gain Your weight may increase gradually over months, or even years, for the onset of myxoedema is insidious. You may not be eating any more than usual, or perhaps you are even eating less, but the pounds gradually accumulate (although large weight gains are uncommon), the increased weight being mainly fluid. Because of this your face may fill out and your facial features become rather blurred – the classical appearance of myxoedema. Hand puffiness is common too.

Thyroid hormone replacement (see Chapter 7) will reduce your weight to your pre-illness level. But I see many overweight people who are convinced that their obesity is due to a thyroid gland problem. Regretfully, this is rarely so – they are just eating too much for their body's current needs, so thyroid replacement treatment is not appropriate.

The weight gain is due to swelling; the classical feature of myxoedema. You may find that you have become somewhat puffy all over and that clothes, glasses, rings and shoes have become tight. Or you may have noticed swelling in the legs particularly; which, by definition, is not supposed to pit, that is, to dent when you prod it gently with your finger. But not every patient reads the textbooks. And some people with myxoedema do have pitting oedema. The swelling is due to leakage of gel-like fluids out of the blood vessels and into the tissues, which in turn hold water in the tissues.

Slow healing and easy bruising You may notice that small cuts take longer to heal because the new skin grows slowly. Or you may be more prone to infections, which can take longer to resolve; this is because you need thyroid hormones for your body's defence mechanisms. Easy bruising is another symptom, due to fragility of the blood vessels.

Brain and Nervous System

Slowing down Slowing down is a very common symptom of myxoedema. As the levels of T3 and T4 fall, your brain gradually slows down. For example, you may notice that you are not doing as much each day as you used to; it may take longer to do jobs or plan things than before; you may think more slowly than you used to; you may be less likely to take the initiative, letting others think for you. Sometimes it is other people – your family or friends – who tell you that you have slowed down.

Tiredness, sleepiness, lack of energy Tiredness is another common, but rather vague, symptom. Lack of thyroid hormone may make you feel generally worn out; the day's work may take so much out of you that you have to have a rest as soon as you get home. Sometimes people with an underactive thyroid fall asleep very easily – at their desks or after lunch, for example. Or it becomes easy to nod off after dinner in the evenings. Rarely, people with severe myxoedema sleep for most of the day. These feelings of tiredness and lack of energy may also combine with the general slowing down.

Getting muddled The brain needs thyroid hormone as much as any other part of the body, so if T3 and T4 levels are low the brain does not work quite as well as it should. This can show itself as minor forgetfulness, or getting muddled over your change when shopping; you may forget people's names or become absent-minded. Rarely, people develop more severe confusion. Children who have lacked thyroid hormone from birth may develop mental retardation or cretinism; early thyroxine treatment completely prevents this tragedy. Modern paediatrics has virtually abolished cretinism.

Depression or other psychiatric symptoms Very rarely, people with myxoedema develop psychiatric symptoms. Sometimes they become depressed; in the old days, people with myxoedema were occasionally labelled as suffering from depression and given psychiatric treatment – as many of the symptoms of myxoedema mimic those of depression, one can understand why. Occasionally, people with myxoedema may temporarily become very disturbed, perhaps believing that their families are trying to poison them, or become very aggressive. Because of this, I believe that every depressed or confused person should have his or her thyroid function checked as a matter of routine; the psychiatric symptoms associated with myxoedema can be completely cured by thyroid replacement therapy, thus obviating the need for psychiatric treatment in such cases.

Incoordination This is a rare symptom. The part of the brain which controls balance and coordination (the cerebellum) can be affected by severe myxoedema, leading to clumsiness, poor balance, with falls in elderly people, trembling hands when reaching out for things, and poor co-ordination. All these settle with treatment.

Numbness and tingling Quite often, people with myxoe-dema may feel numbness, tingling or pins and needles in their hands and feet. This is probably due to pressure on nerves caused by tissue swelling. In the hands, the median nerve can be squashed as it passes through the carpal tunnel at the wrist, causing numbness or tingling in the thumb and first two fingers.

Headaches, coma You may have more headaches than usual, which you will be aware of. And you may even suffer from unconsciousness, which you will not be aware of. Nowadays, fortunately, the latter, known as myxoedema coma, is very uncommon; it may occur in people with myxoedema who get very cold, have a severe infection or accident, or who are short of oxygen. Fits can rarely occur.

Eyes Eye trouble is more often associated with an overactive thyroid gland than an underactive one. However, people can swing from overactive to underactive, and this may affect any eye condition accompanying the initial overactivity (see Chapter 16 for details). In myxoedema the eyelids are often puffy and may be sticky in the morning, needing a lot of rubbing, which can cause soreness. Another cause of sore-ness due to rubbing is watery eyes or epiphora. Occasionally, night vision may be poor.

Ear, Nose and Throat

Hearing You may be troubled by slight deafness. Usually

this simply means that the television sound needs to be turned up a little, although occasionally the hearing impairment is more of a nuisance. There is also a rare inherited condition, with symptoms of white streaks in the hair, underactive thyroid and more severe deafness (Pendred's syndrome).

Snoring People with myxoedema often snore loudly; you are unlikely to notice this yourself, but your partner will. This, combined with falling asleep easily, can lead to some social embarrassment – in the theatre, for example. The increased tendency to snoring is probably due to a thickening of the tissues at the back of the throat. Your tongue may feel large in your mouth.

Hoarse voice Thickening of the vocal cords may cause your voice to become husky. In a few people the voice becomes very hoarse and you sound as if you have a permanent sore throat. Sometimes the voice is deeper, especially in women, or a little slurred.

Swollen neck You may also have a swollen neck caused by a swollen thyroid. This is called a goitre, and can occur in the presence of normal thyroid hormone levels, excess T3 and T4, or in people with myxoedema. See Chapter 17 for a detailed look at goitres.

Digestive System

Poor appetite You may lose your appetite. And it can be very puzzling for a person who is eating less than normal to find themselves putting on weight.

Constipation In myxoedema your bowels slow down, like the rest of your body, and move faeces through the system at a slower rate. This can lead to very stubborn constipation. In

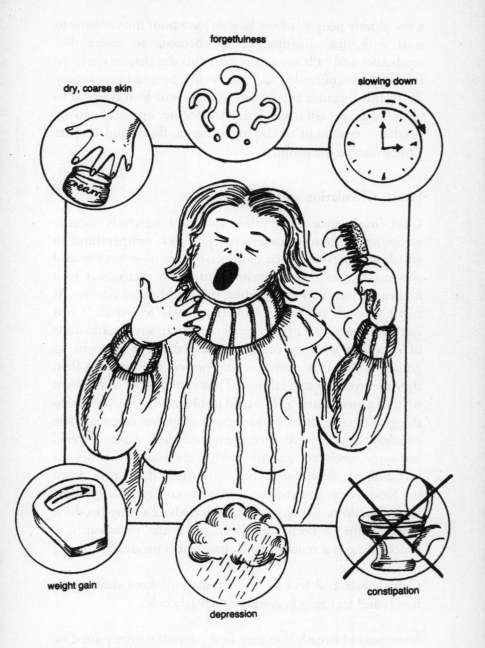

Symptoms of myxoedema.

a few elderly people, whose bowels have poor muscle tone to start with, the constipation can become so severe that medicines and pills are to no avail and the person develops bowel obstruction; they can start vomiting and become very ill. In this instance the person may be sent into hospital to see a surgeon, although it is rare for an operation to be needed – treatment of the myxoedema, fluids and enemas slowly resolve the problem.

Heart, Circulation and Lungs

Cold intolerance Cold intolerance is a relatively specific symptom of thyroid underactivity. Room temperatures in which you previously felt comfortable are now too low and you need extra fires or have to turn the thermostat to a higher setting. You start adding more and more clothes. At night you pile on extra blankets and still feel cold. 'I just can't get warm, doctor' is one of the commonest complaints of a person with myxoedema. Sometimes it happens so gradually that it is a relative who notices the problem first; they are sweating and taking off layers of clothes as you turn up the central heating. The cold intolerance is mainly due to sluggish circulation, for your heart pumps less often and less strongly if you have severe myxoedema. When thyroid hormone levels are low the body's chemical processes, or metabolism, slow down, including those that break down the food we eat and convert it into the energy which powers body functions. These processes release heat as a by-product, which helps to keep you warm, so if the metabolism is functioning at a reduced level, less heat is produced.

Cold hands and feet As the circulation slows down your hands and feet may become particularly cold.

Shortness of breath You may find yourself a little puffed on hills or going upstairs, although severe shortness of breath is rare. This may be due to several factors – fluid accumulation around the lungs, the slow heart rate and less strong heart beat, anaemia and excess weight.

Chest pain Chest pain may also occur, although this is not a symptom of the thyroid underactivity but of its consequences. Lack of T3 and T4 alters fat metabolism (see page 42) and this can lead to furring of the coronary arteries (coronary atherosclerosis) and reduction of blood supply to some of the heart muscle. This causes angina (see page 67) – pain in the chest on exercising, which is usually relieved by rest. Angina is rare in people with myxoedema – call your doctor immediately if you have chest pain.

Blackouts These are an infrequent way for myxoedema to show itself. Like the rest of the body, the heart slows down and the pulse rate may become so slow that the heart stops briefly and then recovers again. This situation may require emergency treatment to help the heart keep beating steadily while thyroid replacement treatment is started. You should see your doctor immediately if you have a blackout.

Bones and Muscles

Weak muscles and stiff joints People with myxoedema often say that their muscles feel weak and stiff, and that they ache. As part of the general slowing up, your muscles may respond very slowly. In addition they may also be slow to return to normal relaxation after a movement, although few people notice this themselves. As a result, it may be hard to do things as vigorously as usual; sportsmen may find a considerable fall in their performance. Walking can become slow and clumsy, especially in cold weather. You may think you have arthritis, with stiff and aching joints. The joints only rarely become swollen, though. Some people may find talking difficult.

Growing Children with severe myxoedema do not grow properly. Fortunately, childhood myxoedema is uncommon nowadays.

Sexual function

Period problems Thyroid hormone lack can cause confusion in other hormone systems. For example, erratic sex hormone production can cause heavy and irregular periods.

Lack of interest in sex You may be too tired for sex, and have a headache, but in addition the interference with sex hormones which occurs can reduce your libido or sexual drive, whether you are a man or a woman.

Infertility If the sex hormones are confused, the ovum may not be released and then the woman cannot conceive; rarely, a man may make insufficient sperm. Some women with myxoedema may stop having periods and may start making breast milk. This is due to a rise in the milk-producing hormone, prolactin, in response to thyroid hormone lack. The prolactin level and symptoms will return to normal with thyroxine treatment. Rarely, a woman with untreated myxoedema may have a miscarriage or stillbirth. Thyroid hormone levels are measured routinely in infertility clinics, for underactivity is readily treatable, allowing a return to normal fertility.

Summary

There are many symptoms of myxoedema, but no one has all of them. They include:

- Changes in appearance such as dry skin, sallow complexion, puffiness, weight gain and swelling.
- Slowing down, tiredness, energy lack and other changes in

thinking or behaviour.
- Ear, nose and throat symptoms include hoarseness and deafness.
- Constipation is a common digestive symptom.
- Cold intolerance is a classical symptom of myxoedema.
- Muscles may become weak, joints stiff and fingers numb.
- There may be problems with periods and sex life.

The symptoms improve with thyroid hormone replacement treatment.

4

Underactive Thyroid – What the Doctor Looks For

All doctors are taught to record your story and to examine you in much the same way; this is so that they obtain all the information they need to help you every time. Of course, they will adjust the questions and examination to suit the condition, but if you understand how your doctor's mind works it will make it easier for you to explain matters and for him to assess you. Try jotting down information before you see the doctor so that you make sure you tell him everything you are worried about.

Your Story

Your doctor will want to know why you have decided to come to see him and what symptoms have been worrying you most. Remember, symptoms are things you have noticed wrong with yourself or unusual feelings. So tell him the most worrying things first, and then the others. Tell him how it all began, from the time you last felt really well, and how it has progressed since then. It helps to know when each symptom started, when it stopped (or if you still have it), what brings it on, what makes it better or worse, and, most of all, exactly what the symptom consists of. For example, contrast 'I feel rather cold, doctor' with 'I always feel cold all over, doctor, even if other people are hot. My hands and feet are especially cold. I've turned the central heating up but I still need extra bedclothes. I first noticed it four months ago, but it's getting worse.'

Once you have told your story, the doctor may ask you some questions to clarify details and to gain further information about related symptoms.

Previous medical history

It is important to tell every new doctor you see about illnesses and operations you have had in the past, or conditions you still have, even if you cannot see how they might influence your current illness. For example, you may have nearly forgotten the bout of rheumatic fever you had 30 years ago when you were 10 years old – surely that's got nothing to do with thyroid trouble? No, it hasn't, but your breathlessness and swollen ankles may be due to heart damage from rheumatic fever rather than fluid retention from myxoedema.

Have you ever had a thyroid operation? Or X-ray treatment to your neck? Have you ever had an overactive thyroid, and, if so, what treatment did you have for it? Did you ever have radioactive iodine treatment? Do you have diabetes or pernicious anaemia?

Family history

As you will see later (pages 46–47), thyroid disease runs in families. Does anyone in your family have an overactive thyroid or an underactive one? Did they in the past? Is there a family history of diabetes or pernicious anaemia?

Your job and lifestyle

Some places, for example, mountainous areas, are associated

with iodine lack and goitre, so your doctor will be interested in where you live now and where you lived before.

Your job and responsibilities are unlikely to have included factors which cause thyroid disease, but it is important that your doctor understands what you do and what it entails mentally and physically. Also, are you responsible for other people's safety? Do you have to make rapid decisions or rely on strong muscles or finely balanced movements?

What sort of person are you? Are you usually the life and soul of the party, but have now slowed down and are a bit miserable because of myxoedema? Or have you always been a quiet, steady person, so that no one noticed you gradually become quieter and start to slow down?

Eating, drinking and smoking As weight gain, despite loss of appetite, is often a symptom of thyroid underactivity, your doctor may want to know how much you usually eat and whether your eating pattern has changed. What sort of foods do you eat? For example, people who eat huge quantities of cabbage are supposed to be more likely to have thyroid swelling or goitres. Do you eat a lot of fatty foods? Your blood cholesterol level is likely to be high until your thyroid underactivity is treated. Drinking excessive alcohol or any smoking at all are both major health hazards, whatever your underlying illness, and smoking is especially hazardous in people with a high cholesterol level.

Drugs and medicines. Allergies Do you take any drugs? By this I don't mean street drugs – although if you have ever taken these you should tell your doctor. I mean any kind of pills, tablets, potions, medicines, injections, unguents, herbal remedies, homoeopathic medicines you may be using. It includes medicines you have bought at the pharmacist's, like aspirin or paracetamol. It is vitally important that you know what you are taking and that you make sure every doctor you see knows what you are taking.

So often, people only tell a particular doctor about the medicines in which they think he is interested. So they will list their blood pressure pills to Dr Jones but omit to mention their heart pills ('I see Dr Brown for that'). Then they wonder why they feel poorly when Dr Jones prescribes new blood-pressure pills (because the new pills do not mix with the heart pills). Some drugs, like aspirin, can interfere with thyroid function tests. And some herbal remedies may contain salicylates (the active ingredient of aspirin) or may contain large quantities of iodine – seaweed pills, for example.

Always tell your doctor if you think you have had a reaction to your medication. And if you have had such a reaction (an allergy or other unwanted effect) to any medication, make sure you know exactly what the proper name of the drug was and what it did to you. The name should be printed on the label of the bottle or on your prescription card. Check with your doctor. Write the name down and then tell every doctor you see what happened.

The rest of your body

Once the details of your story have been checked, the doctor may ask some apparently totally irrelevant questions. These so-called direct questions are to check that the rest of you is all right – your chest, digestive system, urinary system, and so on.

Examination – Looking for Signs

A sign is something your doctor finds when he examines you. For example, if you have myxoedema you may walk slowly into the room and sit down listlessly. Your handshake may be slow to grip and relax, and cold, and your 'Good afternoon' husky or hoarse. You may respond slowly to questions and it may take a long time to work out the answers. You may look sad or very sleepy. You are probably wearing thick sweaters and a coat, despite the warmth of the consulting room.

You may be overweight, and pale with a sallow complexion and sometimes pink/red cheeks. There may be yellow/white fatty deposits on your upper eyelids (called xanthelasmata) and white fatty rings (called corneal arcus) around the iris of the eye (the coloured bit). Your face, especially the eyelids, may be puffy. Other puffy areas might include the hands (especially the backs), and the tops of the feet. Your skin may look dry and flaky, with areas of thick dry skin on pressure points like the elbows and heels. You may have bruises. Your nails may be white, dry and broken and the hair thin and lacklustre. The outer third of the eyebrows may be thin or missing.

Your doctor will be able to observe all of these signs without touching you; indeed, they may be sufficient to make the diagnosis clinically. Your skin may feel cold and dry to the touch. Anaemia may be diagnosed by looking at the pallor of the hands and the lower eyelids. The tongue may appear full. You may have an obvious thyroid swelling – or it may not be possible to feel the thyroid gland at all.

Heart, circulation and lungs

A slow pulse is characteristic of myxoedema (a slow pulse is called bradycardia). Your hands and feet may have reduced circulation, although the main pulses can be readily felt. Your blood pressure may be low or normal. In severe myxoedema the heart may be enlarged due to fluid around it – called pericardial effusion – but this is rare. If the heart has been severely weakened by lack of thyroid hormone, there may be heart failure, with pitting swelling of feet and ankles.

The lungs The lungs are rarely affected by myxoedema, but occasionally fluid surrounds them and this can be detected by your doctor, who will tap your chest with his fingers and listen to your breathing.

The abdomen The abdomen often feels doughy and dry. Your internal organs will usually be normal, but your doctor may feel the fullness and lumpiness of your bowel if you have severe constipation. If the constipation has been very troublesome or caused you abdominal pain he may perform a rectal examination by gently inserting a lubricated gloved finger into the rectum. This does not hurt but is just slightly uncomfortable and may make you feel as if you want to open your bowels. Some men may develop scrotal swelling if fluid accumulates there. This is called hydrocele and is not serious.

Nervous system including vision and hearing

Daytime vision is usually normal, unless thyroid eye disease has caused problems (see pages 133–139). But your hearing may be reduced; to check it your doctor may ask you to listen to a tuning fork. If you have complained of weak muscles he may test your strength, looking at each limb in turn. It is also important to check your tendon reflexes by tapping the elbows, wrists, knees and ankles with a small tendon hammer. Classically the reflex jerks relax slowly in myxoedema. A few hospitals have machines that you kneel beside which measure the relaxation time of the tendon reflex at the ankle.

If you have noticed numbness, pins and needles or tingling, the doctor will ask you exactly where the problem is, and may then touch the skin lightly with cotton wool or a clean pin to check sensation. Tapping over the carpal tunnel at the wrist can sometimes reproduce tingling, due to median nerve compression there. Another name for this is carpal tunnel syndrome (see page 19).

In the few people with myxoedema who have noticed

balance or coordination problems, the doctor will probably check how well you can point to things and how dextrous your fingers are. He may also ask you to walk heel-to-toe to check your balance.

Case History of Myxoedema

John Green is a 58-year-old taxi driver, who has lived in London all his life. This is his case history as written down by a doctor.

Patient complains

- 'I'm tired all the time.'
- 'I keep falling asleep.'
- 'I feel the cold, even in summer.'

History of presenting complaint

For the past six months Mr Green has been excessively tired and fallen asleep readily, both at home and at work. Once he fell asleep in his cab while waiting in a traffic jam. Although previously a 'night-owl', he now goes to bed at 8 p.m. He feels exhausted all the time and has little energy. He has marked cold intolerance and wears extra clothes day and night. His hands and feet are particularly cold, and he now wears gloves for driving, although he never did so previously.

On direct questioning, Mr Green cannot concentrate and finds it hard to calculate the change for customers. He knows London well after 30 years' taxi-driving but has recently got lost on several occasions. He has gained about five pounds in weight but thinks his appetite is normal. He has had increasing constipation for four months, opening his bowels once every three or four days, compared with daily before. The motions are hard but normal in colour. He has dry skin, but thinks his face and hair have not changed.

Previous medical history

- No tuberculosis, rheumatic fever, diabetes, kidney disease or epilepsy.
- Appendicectomy in childhood.
- Right inguinal hernia repair 1978.

Social history

- Mr Green initially planned an army career, but left the army to become a taxi-driver.
- He now has his own terraced house.
- His main hobby is building model railways.
- He gets little exercise.
- His diet consists of snacks during the day, with a high fat and sugar content and little fibre. He has a 'meat and two veg' evening meal.
- He smokes 20 cigarettes a day.
- He drinks two to three pints of beer a week at weekends.

Family history

Mr Green is married with six children. His uncle had an underactive thyroid, his father died from a heart attack aged 75 and his mother is well.

Drugs

- Aspirin, taken occasionally for headaches.
- Senna laxative, for the past four months only.

Allergies

- Penicillin causes rash.

Direct questions

- *Cardiovascular and respiratory system:*
  Smoker's cough producing clear sputum but no blood.
  Short of breath on hills, especially over the past six
  months.
  No chest pain, no palpitations.
  Mild ankle swelling, duration?
- *Gastrointestinal system:*
  Appetite normal, but weight rising.
  No nausea or vomiting.
  No indigestion or abdominal pain.
  Constipation as above.
- *Genito-urinary system:*
  No painful urination or frequency.
  No nocturnal urination.
  No blood.
- *Nervous system:*
  Vague headaches with no obvious precipitating or
  relieving factors apart from aspirin.
  No fits, faints or falls.
  Vision normal with glasses.
  Hearing normal.
  No pins and needles or numbness.
  No muscle weakness.

On examination

- Height 5 foot 10 inches (1.78 metres).
- Weight 13 stone 6 pounds (85.4 kg) (ideal weight
  10 stone to 12 stone 4 lb – 64–79 kg).
- Pale but not anaemic.
- Not cyanosed (blue), jaundiced (yellow).
- No xanthalesmata (fatty spots).
- Full face with puffy eyelids and watery eyes.
- Dry skin, normal hair and nails.

- Nicotine-stained fingers.
- Thyroid impalpable (not felt).

Cardiovascular system

- Pulse 60 beats/minute, regular rhythm.
- Blood pressure 130/88.
- No venous engorgement.
- Apex beat normal position (i.e. heart not enlarged), normal character.
- Heart sounds normal.
- Peripheral pulses full.
- Varicose veins both legs.
- Non-pitting oedema of both feet and ankles.

Respiratory system

- Intermittent cough with white sputum.
- Trachea central.
- Chest expansion normal.
- Percussion (tapping) note normal and equal.
- Breath sounds normal, with added wheezes.
- Chest resonance normal.

Abdomen

- Overweight.
- Appendicectomy and right inguinal hernia repair scars.
- Doughy.
- No enlargement of liver, spleen, kidneys.
- Normal bowel sounds.
- Rectal examination – normal.

Nervous system

- Cranial nerves normal, including hearing and vision.

- Retinae (back of eyes) normal.
- Power, tone, coordination and sensation normal in all limbs.
- Reflexes present, equal, slow-relaxing.

Diagnosis

Myxoedema.

The next section of the case notes would consider confirmatory investigations and health checks, followed by treatment and general health advice. These are considered in Chapters 5 and 7.

What advice would you give Mr Green?

Summary

- Doctors are taught to assess patients in a standardised way – your main symptoms, previous medical history, family and social history, medications, allergies, smoking, alcohol, diet, general questions, clinical examination.
- Clinical examination of someone with myxoedema may reveal slowness, cold dry skin, swelling, overweight, slow pulse and slowly relaxing tendon reflexes.
- There may be no convincing abnormalities on examination.

5

Underactive Thyroid – Tests

In many cases the combination of some of the symptoms and signs detailed in Chapters 3 and 4 allow a doctor to make a confident diagnosis of myxoedema. But it is important to confirm the diagnosis by doing thyroid function tests.

Laboratory Tests for Myxoedema

The doctor or phlebotomist (the person who takes your blood) will take a small sample of blood from a vein, label it carefully and send it, with an accompanying named card, to the laboratory. The laboratory will then spin down the blood in a centrifuge, separating the blood cells from the straw-coloured plasma they are normally suspended in. Other laboratories may allow the blood to clot and then use the clear serum. It is this plasma or serum that is then analysed in the various tests. The thyroid function tests performed by different laboratories vary, both in the methods used and their specificity. It is therefore important for each doctor to know which tests his local laboratory uses and what the local normal ranges are.

Normal thyroid hormone concentrations

Free T4   9–22.7 picomols/1

Free T3	3.5–6.5 picomols/1
Total T4	70–140 nanomols/1
Total T3	1–3 nanomols/1
TSH	0.35–5.0 milliunits/1

n.b. Each laboratory has its own range which may change if they change the assay method.

Free hormone concentrations

The tests which are easiest to interpret are free T4 (thyroxine) and/or free T3 (tri-iodothyronine) along with TSH (thyroid stimulating hormone) assay. This means that, in most cases, the doctor does not have to allow for alterations in the levels of the carrier proteins associated with these hormones (see pages 10–11). If the thyroid is unable to make thyroid hormones, the plasma concentrations, i.e. the concentrations of the hormones circulating in the bloodstream, will fall as the stores in the colloid in the follicles (page 5) are depleted and not replenished. As the blood T3 and T4 concentrations fall, the pituitary gland releases TSH (thyroid stimulating hormone) to encourage increased hormone production in the thyroid gland. This means that the plasma or serum TSH levels rise. When John Green's blood was analysed by the laboratory his thyroid function tests looked like this:

- Free T4, 3 picomol/1.
- Free T3, 1 picomol/1.
- TSH, 45 milliunit/1.

Total thyroid hormone concentrations

Other laboratories use total T3 and T4 tests that measure the carrier protein levels as well. However, many factors can interfere with the interpretation of total thyroid hormone

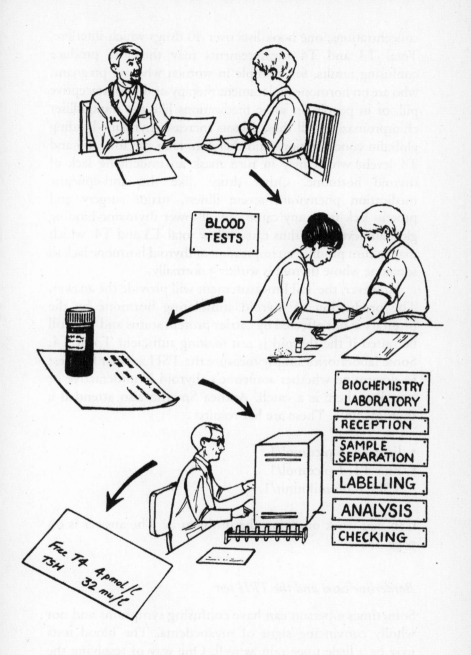

BLOOD
TESTS

BIOCHEMISTRY
LABORATORY

RECEPTION

SAMPLE
SEPARATION

LABELLING

ANALYSIS

CHECKING

Free T4   4 pmol/L
TSH   32 mu/L

Testing for myxoedema.

concentrations; one book lists over 40 drugs which interfere. Total T3 and T4 measurements may therefore produce confusing results, for example in women who are pregnant, who are on hormone replacement therapy or the contraceptive pill, or in people on some medications like the tranquilliser chlorpromazine. All these factors increase thyroxine-binding globulin concentrations and therefore raise the total T3 and T4 levels, which may in turn mask an underlying lack of thyroid hormone. Other drugs, like the anti-epileptic medication phenytoin, severe illness, major surgery and protein lack from any cause can all lower thyroxine-binding globulin levels and thus cause a low total T3 and T4, which may in turn produce an impression of thyroid hormone lack in someone whose thyroid is working normally.

However, the TSH measurement will provide the answer. The production of thyroid stimulating hormone by the pituitary is not affected by carrier protein status and will still be raised if the thyroid is not making sufficient T3 or T4. Some laboratories simply measure the TSH as their first test to determine whether someone's thyroid is underactive or not. But there is a catch. Anthea Smythe also attended a thyroid clinic. These are her results:

- Free T4, 5 picomol/1.
- Free T1, 1 picomol/1.
- TSH, 0.06 milliunit/1.

Can you work out what the problem is? The answer is on page 53.

Borderline cases and the TRH test

Sometimes a person can have confusing symptoms and not wholly convincing signs of myxoedema. The blood tests may be a little uncertain as well. One way of resolving the problem is to wait a few months and then see what happens;

the situation will usually become more obvious on sub-sequent examination and tests. This is a practical course of action, for no doctor would wish to start what is probably life-long treatment without convincing evidence that it is needed. However, it may mean that the person who really is becoming hypothyroid feels below par for longer than necessary (see page 47 for further discussion).

One solution to the borderline problem is to see how the pituitary gland responds to stimulation. If concentrations of T3 and T4 are indeed lower than normal, then the pituitary gland will have responded by making and storing more TSH (thyroid stimulating hormone) than usual. If this is the case, an injection of TRH (thyrotrophin releasing hormone, normally made in the hypothalamus, see page 10) will then make the pituitary release its stores of TSH in a great whoosh, producing TSH levels of 20 milliunit/1 or more in men, 25 milliunit/1 or more in women, within 20 minutes after injection. In contrast, the normal response shows a smaller rise than this. And if the pituitary gland is not working at all there will be no rise in TSH.

TRH may sometimes make people feel hot and produce a tingling sensation in the genital area. This is a normal and harmless effect, but people with epilepsy should not be given TRH as it may cause a fit in people prone to this.

Thyroid antibodies

An antibody is a chemical produced by the white blood cells in response to any chemical trigger which the body perceives as a threat. Such chemical triggers are called antigens, and the antibody binds with the antigen and immobilises it. This is called an immune reaction; it is how we defend ourselves from infection. If you cannot produce antibodies you are at risk from infection – this is what happens in acquired immune deficiency syndrome (AIDS), and in some other conditions in which antibody production fails.

However, more frequently the opposite problem arises – unnecessary antibodies are produced. The body gets confused and starts to produce antibodies against a part of itself, i.e. it behaves as if one of its own chemicals is a threat. This process is called autoimmunity, and is nothing whatsoever to do with AIDS.

In thyroid disorders the white blood cells make antibodies against parts of the thyroid gland. The autoantibodies that most laboratories measure are those that bind to microsomes – tiny particles inside the thyroid cells. These autoantibodies are called thyroid microsomal antibodies, while those against thyroglobulin (see pages 5–8) are called thyroglobulin antibodies.

The presence of thyroid microsomal or thyroglobulin antibodies does not in itself mean that you are hypothyroid, but it does provide supporting evidence, in conjunction with the clinical picture and other blood tests (see page 47).

Other Tests

Blood count

About one in four people with an underactive thyroid develop anaemia – the body makes fewer blood cells because of the slowed metabolism. This resolves once the thyroid hormone levels return to normal.

Blood cholesterol concentration

One in two people in the United Kingdom have a blood cholesterol level which is above desirable limits. Myxoedema causes the cholesterol level to rise, probably because it is not cleared from the body as efficiently as usual, although other chemical mechanisms contribute to the process. Before thyroid hormone concentrations could be assayed directly, doctors used to measure cholesterol to support the diagnosis of myxoedema. Provided you do not have an underlying cholesterol problem, your cholesterol level will return to normal with thyroid replacement treatment.

Blood urea and electrolyte concentrations

Electrolytes are chemicals such as sodium and potassium, and are essential for normal body energy and fluid balance. In myxoedema the blood sodium level may be low because less water is cleared from the body than normal, which in turn dilutes the sodium carried in the blood. Rarely, the blood potassium may be high, although this occurs if you have adrenal insufficiency as well, the latter being an uncommon problem. Adrenal hormone lack can also lower the blood concentration of urea, one of the body's waste products (see page 152).

Glucose

The blood glucose level will be normal in myxoedema. However, diabetes may occur in hypothyroid people (and vice versa), in which case the blood glucose will be raised. It is important to check this, as it will need treatment (see page 150).

Electrocardiogram

This is an electrical recording of the heart's activity, often abbreviated to ECG (EKG in America). The tiny electrical signals produced by the heart as it beats are recorded by sensors placed on the chest and limbs. Usually the ECG simply shows a slow pulse, but it may also show other changes, suggesting that parts of the heart are not getting enough blood because their blood vessels are narrowed by fatty deposits.

Summary

- The clinical diagnosis of myxoedema is confirmed by measuring low concentrations of the thyroid hormones T3 and T4, in the blood.
- The TSH level is usually raised, unless the pituitary gland is not making it.
- Different laboratories use different assay methods and have different normal ranges.
- TRH will produce an exaggerated TSH response in myxoedema.
- The blood tests have to be interpreted in the light of the clinical picture and within the limitations of the tests.

6

Underactive Thyroid – Causes

At some time or another everyone who becomes ill asks themselves the same question – 'Why me?' Thyroid underactivity is common especially in women, who are affected about 10 times more often than men. Three out of every 100 women have myxoedema and four in every 1,000 women will develop new myxoedema each year. One in 2,000 men will develop new myxoedema each year.

Causes of myxoedema

Common causes (in the UK)

Autoimmune thyroiditis (Hashimoto's thyroiditis) – about 70 per cent.

Previous treatment for thyrotoxicosis – about 20 per cent.

Uncommon causes

Iodine deficiency (common in other countries).
Drugs – lithium, amiodarone.
Pituitary damage.
Hypothalamic damage.
Inability to use thyroid hormone (tissue resistance).
Congenitally absent or abnormal thyroid.
Inability to make normal thyroid hormones.

Autoimmune Thyroid Disorders

Autoimmune conditions are those in which the body's own (*auto* means self) defence mechanism, the immune system, attacks part of the body, under the mistaken impression that it is destroying a potentially harmful invader (see page 150). The tendency of this to happen can be inherited, which is why doctors ask for details of your family history.

Tissues which are particularly likely to be affected by an autoimmune process are the thyroid, the pancreas (causing diabetes), the stomach (preventing absorption of vitamin B12 and causing pernicious anaemia), the joints (causing rheumatoid arthritis) and the adrenal glands (causing Addison's disease or adrenal insufficiency). If you have one autoimmune disorder you are more likely than the population as a whole to have others. The commonest such link is between diabetes and thyroid disease; indeed, some doctors test all new patients with diabetes for thyroid disease, and many test all new patients with overactive or underactive thyroids for diabetes (see page 150).

Some people with myxoedema inherit the tendency for chemicals on or in their thyroid cells to act as antigens, i.e. to provoke an autoimmune response; perhaps some outside event activates these antigens, allowing them to trigger the body's defence mechanisms. The antigens are detected by white blood cells called lymphocytes. There are several sorts of lymphocyte circulating in the bloodstream and some lymphocytes make antibodies targeted against various parts of the thyroid gland. Up to one in five people with myxoedema have antibodies which block the TSH receptors (see page 10) on the surface of thyroid cells. If these receptors are blocked, the TSH produced by the pituitary cannot stimulate thyroid hormone production. Most of the antibodies which attack the thyroid can only be measured in research laboratories; however, microsomal and thyroglobulin antibodies (see page 42) are two which can be measured routinely.

In some cases the autoimmune response is such that lymphocytes swarm into the thyroid gland and produce antibodies that attack the thyroid cells and destroy them. This condition is sometimes called Hashimoto's disease. In some forms of attack the thyroid tissue is replaced by lymphocytes; in others there are islands of normal follicles and islands of lymphocytes. Eventually, though, after a severe attack, the whole thyroid is destroyed and is replaced by inactive fibrous tissue like a scar.

It is thought that a person inherits the vulnerability to this sort of autoimmune attack – or that they inherit lack of protection from attack. The attack is probably triggered by one or several environmental factors such as infection, dietary factors, injury, smoking, chemicals, drugs and stress. However, it is possible (although less likely) that the antibodies that we can measure are in fact produced as a result of some earlier attack on the thyroid, by a different mechanism. Furthermore, there are other factors such as your gender (women are much more likely to have auto-immune thyroid disease than men), your hormone status and how old you are.

Premyxoedema, borderline myxoedema or subclinical hypothyroidism

Some doctors in north-east England (The Whickham Survey) measured thyroid antibodies in a cross-section of the population there. They found that between 2 and 4 per cent of men and 8 and 15 per cent of women had antibodies to thyroid tissue in their blood, thyroid antibodies being commonest in women over 40 years old; the average was about three out of every 100 men and eight out of every 100 women. They also found that about four in every 100 men and 12 out of every 100 women had a raised TSH level. This suggested that thyroid underactivity was very much more common than was apparent from the numbers of people actually receiving treatment for it. If there are a lot of people with thyroid antibodies and a high TSH who have not felt ill enough to contact their doctors, should we be screening the whole population for myxoedema, all over the country?

Some centres have tried this. The problem is that when we actually find the people with thyroid antibodies and a high TSH, they may well have no symptoms at all and no abnormalities on examination. Furthermore, the free T3 and T4 levels in their bloodstream may be normal. We can do a TRH test (page 40), which often shows an exaggerated response, and this has led to the concept of premyxoedema or subclinical hypothyroidism.

Various groups of doctors and scientists have studied this problem. The north-eastern group (and others) found that, out of 100 women with thyroid antibodies and high TSH, five will develop obvious thyroid underactivity each year. If we extend this calculation (which may not produce a completely accurate answer, for other factors are involved), by the end of 20 years all the women would have underactive thyroids.

There is debate as to the best management of this situation. If the TSH is raised and you have thyroid antibodies you will eventually develop an underactive thyroid gland. Therefore my personal view is that if your TSH is raised in two separate samples you should start 25 micrograms of thyroxine daily to be increased to the dose which returns the TSH to within normal range.

If your TSH is above normal without thyroid antibodies I would suggest six monthly review. However, some other doctors would treat anyone with a TSH over 2 milliunits/l who had symptoms of hypothyroidism unexplained by any other cause.

Sometimes, I may start someone with a raised TSH (with or without antibodies) on thyroxine if they have a raised cholesterol which does not have another obvious cause (see page 42).

Whatever the follow up arrangements you agree with your doctor, contact him earlier if you develop any of the symptoms of an underactive thyroid or if you are planning pregnancy (see page 125).

I should emphasise that this is just one person's view and that there are other, equally valid views on management. However, most doctors would agree that a person with raised TSH and thyroid antibodies should have regular i.e. at least annual, checks to detect the onset of symptoms or signs of myxoedema or a fall in free T4.

Treatment for Thyroid Overactivity

It is estimated that about one in three people with myxoedema have had surgical or radioiodine treatment for thyroid overactivity in the past.

Thyroid surgery

If you have had an operation to remove part of your thyroid gland in the past you are more likely than other people to develop thyroid underactivity later. The answer seems simple – there is not quite enough thyroid tissue to provide all the thyroid hormones you need. In fact it is a little more complicated, as most people who have had part of their thyroid removed have the operation to treat an overactive thyroid gland. People with thyroid overactivity may also have thyroglobulin and microsomal antibodies, which increase their likelihood of developing thyroid underactivity whether or not part of the thyroid gland is removed. Between one and eight in ten people who have had thyroid surgery will develop myxoedema.

Radioactive iodine treatment

This is mainly used to treat thyroid overactivity. Radioactive iodine (also called radioiodine or I^{131} treatment, because that is the radioactive version of iodine used) carries a very high risk of thyroid underactivity (see page 115).

Inflammation of the Thyroid Gland

Viruses can cause inflammation of the thyroid gland, just as they can cause inflammation elsewhere in the body. This is called thyroiditis (-*itis* means inflammation). There are several names for this condition – one version is called de Quervain's thyroiditis. Hashimoto's disease is a form of autoimmune thyroiditis.

Viral thyroiditis can cause painful and very tender swelling of the thyroid, the illness perhaps starting rather like an ordinary cough or cold. Initially, the inflamed follicles may release lots of T3 and T4 into the bloodstream and cause a temporary thyroid overactivity. Then the thyroid may become underactive until the inflammation has settled and the follicular cells have recovered.

Thyroiditis can be a temporary cause of thyroid insufficiency, requiring short-term treatment only. Hashimoto's thyroiditis (page 47) can cause long-term myxoedema.

Drugs

Lithium is used to treat psychiatric conditions such as manic-depressive illnesses. It interferes with the manufacture of thyroid hormones and reduces their release into the circulation. About half the patients on long-term lithium treatment have a goitre and one in five develops myxoedema. People taking lithium should have their thyroid function tested every three months. Rarely, lithium has been associated with thyrotoxicosis.

Amiodarone is used to control severe abnormalities of heart rhythm. It contains iodine and can reduce the release of thyroid hormones from the thyroid. Amiodarone also blocks conversion of T4 to T3 in the body tissues. Because it contains iodine, it can also cause thyroid overactivity which can be difficult to control. It takes a long time to clear from the body.

Iodine

Iodine deficiency is the commonest cause of myxoedema throughout the world, and is mainly found in mountainous areas like the Himalayas, Andes and Alps.

Lack of iodine means that the thyroid gland cannot produce T4 and T3. This triggers the pituitary gland to produce TSH, but without iodine even TSH stimulation cannot increase T3 and T4 production. The thyroid swells as the number of cells inside it increases as a result of the TSH stimulation, and the person develops a goitre.

Iodine deficiency is no longer the main cause of myxoedema in the United Kingdom – iodised table salt is all that is needed to correct such a lack of dietary iodine in geographically deficient areas. However, you may still hear people talk about Derbyshire neck, describing the goitres previously common in this iodine-deficient area.

Iodine excess

Iodine has very complex effects on the thyroid. Large doses of iodine taken over a few days actually block thyroid hormone production by upsetting the balance of the chemical reactions which incorporate iodine into T3 and T4. This effect can be useful in the acute treatment of an overactive thyroid (see page 108).

If you eat too much iodine over a long time, for example from seaweed-derived remedies or from iodized cough sweets, this too can block the production of thyroid hormones in some people whose chemical pathways are not quite normal. These people can also develop thyroid swelling or goitre. In others excess iodine causes thyrotoxicosis (see page 99).

Congenital Myxoedema (also known as endemic cretinism)

This means thyroid underactivity you are born with, and it occurs in about one in 4,000 newborn babies. World-wide between five and 15 percent of the population may be born with thyroid underactivity. There are several causes but the commonest is absence or abnormal development of the thyroid gland. Rarer causes include failures in the chemical sequence in which thyroid hormones are made. Untreated, congenital myxoedema causes severe physical and mental disability.

Pituitary Gland Problems

All the causes of myxoedema described so far have been due to problems within the thyroid gland itself. But occasionally the thyroid factory can be capable of working well but be unable to produce the goods because of problems at the pituitary head office. You will remember Anthea Smythe's laboratory results on page 40.

Case History

Anthea Smythe was 41 years old when she went to see her doctor because she had had no periods for a year. Her periods had been regular until about three years ago and it seemed rather early for the change of life. Milk had begun to leak from her breasts on occasions, even though she had not had a baby for 10 years. Indeed, she had been sterilised, so she was certain she could not be pregnant now. She had also noticed that she felt the cold severely. Her muscles ached and seemed weak. She had started to feel dizzy when she stood up suddenly. Her husband thought she looked very pale.

On examination, Anthea's doctor noted that she did look pale and her skin seemed smooth. Her face was puffy, especially around the eyes, and her pale cold hands and feet were puffy too. She seemed very weary, and admitted that she had been feeling tired and under the weather recently. Anthea had a pulse rate of 58 beats per minute (which is slow) and her blood pressure was 105/60 lying down, falling to 90/45 on standing, when she also felt dizzy. Milk could be expressed from both nipples, which were pale. She had very little underarm or pubic hair. Pelvic examination was normal. Neurological examination was normal, except for slow relaxation of her tendon reflexes.

If you look through Anthea's symptoms and signs, you will recognise some of the features of myxoedema. But not all of the findings can be explained by thyroid trouble alone. It is very rare for myxoedema to cause the breasts to make milk. One would not expect someone with myxoedema to lose their body hair. And although people with myxoedema can have a low blood pressure, severe postural hypotension (fall in blood pressure on standing) is unusual. So her doctor tested her blood – her thyroid function tests were:

- Free T4 5 picomol/1.
- Free T3 1 picomol/1.
- TSH 0.06 milliunit/1.

Her thyroid was obviously underactive, as indicated by the low free T4 and free T3, but the TSH level was low too. That showed that the pituitary gland had been unable to respond to the low T3 and T4 levels – it showed, in fact, that the cause of the problem was not in the thyroid gland at all but in the pituitary gland. Further tests on Anthea's blood showed that levels of pituitary sex hormones were low, explaining her loss of body hair, and that Anthea was making insufficient steroid hormones, explaining why her blood pressure fell on standing. She was also making enormous quantities of the milk-producing hormone, prolactin.

A special X-ray, a CT (computed tomography) scan, showed that there was a large tumour in her pituitary gland. The tumour was removed surgically through her nose and shown to be made of prolactin-producing cells. It was benign – it is exceedingly rare to find cancer in the pituitary gland – but it had squashed the cells making the pituitary hormones controlling sex hormone and adrenal steroid production, and also those making TSH.

Anthea Smythe had an uncommon but readily treat-able problem. She is now completely well on full replace-ment treatment – thyroxine, steroids and sex hormones, the steroid hormones being started first so that her body could cope with the increase in her metabolism caused by the thyroxine. The only sign of the pituitary operation is a tiny scar on her lip. Looking back, Anthea thinks she had been feeling ill for at least three years.

Hypothalamic Problems

You will recall that the thyroid 'factory' is controlled by the pituitary 'head office' and that the pituitary is in turn controlled by the hypothalamus 'managing director' (see page 10) – it is the hypothalamus that makes TSH releasing hormone (TRH).

Extremely rarely, problems in the hypothalamus, for example cysts, can cause a deficiency of TRH, so TSH is not made by the pituitary and hence T4 and T3 are not made by the thyroid.

Summary

- Thyroid underactivity is common.
- The commonest cause of myxoedema in the United Kingdom is autoimmune thyroid disease. Many people have antibodies to thyroid tissue, but not all of them have myxoedema.
- Other causes are thyroid surgery and radioactive iodine, both usually originally used to treat an overactive thyroid gland.
- Worldwide iodine deficiency is the commonest cause of myxoedema. This can be corrected by everyone in iodine-deficient areas using iodised salt.
- Sometimes too much iodine can cause myxoedema too.
- Temporary myxoedema may occur with inflammation of the thyroid, thyroiditis, and during or after pregnancy.
- Rarely, the pituitary gland stops making TSH, or, very rarely, the hypothalamus stops making TRH. This causes myxoedema too. There may be deficiencies in other hormones in this situation.

7
Underactive Thyroid – Treatment

Thyroid Hormone Replacement

Just over 100 years ago Murray and his colleagues first showed that thyroid extract could cure myxoedema. Nowadays pure thyroxine is used, or, rarely, tri-iodothyronine. The dose of thyroxine ranges from 25 micrograms to 300 micrograms, 25 micrograms often being too little to have much effect and few people needing as much as 300 micrograms. The standard maintenance dose is 100 to 150 micrograms once a day. Treatment is usually for life, but as thyroxine is simply a natural hormone which replaces what is missing it has no side effects, other than those of too large or too small a dose.

Starting thyroxine replacement

Thyroxine therapy should always be started gradually so that the body becomes used to it; too much thyroxine, too early, may speed up the metabolism too much. The usual starting dose of thyroxine is 50 to 100 micrograms daily. Many doctors would start with 50 micrograms. See your doctor after about six weeks of treatment to review your symptoms and to check thyroid hormone levels. Elderly people should probably start on 25 micrograms a day.

People with heart problems The speeding up of the body and the heart rate produced by thyroxine replacement causes an extra demand on the heart. In the few people with coronary atherosclerosis (furring-up of the blood vessels supplying oxygen and nutrients to the heart muscle) some areas of heart muscle may not get enough blood, which can worsen angina or cause a heart attack or coronary thrombosis. If you have had previous heart trouble, suffer from angina or have an abnormal ECG, some doctors would start you on 25 micrograms of thyroxine a day for three to four weeks, under careful supervision, often in hospital. They may increase your anti-angina treatment such as beta-blocker pills (like propranolol). Other doctors would admit you to hospital and start you on a small dose of tri-iodothyronine, changing to thyroxine later. The dose of thyroxine will then be increased very cautiously according to how you respond. If you have any chest pains after starting thyroxine treatment you must contact your doctor straightaway.

Transient myxoedema This is not common but treatment should be sought. Pregnancy is one cause (see page 127). Transient thyroid insufficiency can also occur after thyroid surgery such as subtotal thyroidectomy (see page 116–118) or after radioactive iodine treatment (see page 110) for thyroid overactivity. It is unusual for such patients to manage without thyroxine long term. If your myxoedema is pregnancy related or follows thyroid surgery or radioiodine and you need only a small dose of thyroxine to maintain normal thyroid hormone levels, it is worth stopping the thyroxine after three to six months and retesting thyroid function four to six weeks later.

In general, if you are uncertain as to whether you really need thyroxine replacement or not, ask your doctor about a trial without tablets followed by a reassessment at four to six weeks. Do *not* do this without talking to your doctor – I have seen a patient so ill that she could not walk after stopping essential thyroxine replacement.

Maintenance thyroxine treatment

Once you are well established on treatment it is important to have just the right amount of thyroxine on a long-term basis. Too much and you will develop the features of thyroid overactivity. Too little and you will remain myxoedematous. But one of the problems in deciding the right dose is that different tissues in the body seem to recover from myxoedema at different rates. Furthermore, it may take six months or longer for the symptoms to resolve completely.

Talk to your doctor. How do you feel? Have your symptoms resolved? Or at least, have they improved? To back up your own impressions, your doctor can weigh you, measure your pulse rate, look at your facial appearance, your skin, the tissue swelling or myxoedema.

Thyroid function tests can help but should not be regarded as the sole indicator of treatment balance. The TSH level should have returned to within the normal range as this reflects the thyroid hormone levels as 'perceived' by one tissue (the pituitary). The free T4 level itself should be within the normal range, although this is less helpful than it might at first seem as it simply shows that the pills you are swallowing are being absorbed. The free T3 level might perhaps be more helpful as this is the active form of thyroid hormone, but is harder to measure for most laboratories. The free T3 level should be within the normal range. It is important not to over-treat myxoedema as this will cause the same problems as thyrotoxicosis (see Chapter 9). Your cholesterol will return to normal with adequate thyroxine treatment – unless you have an underlying cholesterol problem. Have a thyroid function test every year for life.

Tri-iodothyronine treatment

This treatment can be used in the very few people who cannot absorb thyroxine, or in people who can take nothing by mouth. It can be given by intravenous injection.

It is shorter-acting than thyroxine, a property which can in itself be useful in starting treatment in people with very severe myxoedema or heart trouble.

Occasionally, people ask to change to tri-iodothyronine treatment because they have heard it is 'better' than thyroxine. This is unlikely to be the case. In people with normal thyroid function, most of the thyroid hormone circulating in their blood is T4 (thyroxine) and the body tissues convert this to T3 (tri-iodothyronine) as required. The pituitary relies on T4 for half its TSH regulation, so giving sufficient tri-iodothyronine tablets to suppress TSH might actually provide an overdose of T3 in other body tissues.

Iodine Treatment

Few people in Britain today have dietary iodine deficiency. In most areas of iodine deficiency people are now encouraged to use iodised salt. If you know your diet is iodine deficient you should discuss iodine supplements with your doctor.

Once someone has developed an underactive thyroid gland they need thyroxine replacement treatment. But do not be tempted to add to your doctor's thyroid treatment by buying herbal or health-shop remedies like kelp or other iodine-containing supplements merely because the label claims they are 'good for the thyroid'. (Some cough remedies also contain iodine, so check the label.) It is not a good idea to overdo your iodine intake as this has unpredictable effects (see page 51).

Keeping Healthy Generally

Obviously thyroxine replacement treatment is the most important factor in helping you to recover from your myxoedema. But you must also keep yourself as healthy as possible generally to regain full fitness.

Diet

Although many people with myxoedema are overweight, this is mostly fluid and will disappear as the thyroxine treatment takes effect. However, if you were overweight before your thyroid gland slowed down, you will still need to do something about this problem. Because of the myxoedema your cholesterol level will also probably be high. This too will resolve, unless you have an underlying tendency to high cholesterol. However, while your body is sorting itself out under the thyroxine treatment, start looking at the sorts of foods you are eating, and their quantities. The constipation that often develops in myx-oedematous people is another factor that you ought to consider. Your diet is what you eat. A healthy diet should contain lots of high-fibre starchy carbohydrate foods such as wholemeal bread, potatoes in their jackets, beans, pulses and oat bran; but little sugary carbohydrate food like sweets, candies, chocolate, biscuits, cookies and plain sugar. Your diet should be especially low in animal fats like butter, cream, hard cheese or fatty meat. And if you were overweight before you became myxoedematous, do not eat too much as your appetite returns. If you are constipated eat plenty of soft fruit and vegetables.

Smoking

Smoking kills one in two smokers – it is so dangerous that you should stop immediately. Smoking is more addictive than heroin, so it can be very hard to give up your cigarettes. However, most people find it less hard to stop smoking altogether than to try to reduce gradually.

If your thyroid is underactive you are already at increased risk of coronary atherosclerosis – heart disease. And heart disease is a major risk of cigarette smoking; it is rare to see a non-smoker as a patient in a coronary care unit. So people who have an underactive thyroid gland should not smoke – it considerably increases your likelihood of having a heart attack.

Exercise

If your thyroid gland has been underactive for some time your muscles may well be weak and stiff, and they may ache. They will certainly take time to recover. To help them recover their tone and strength, discuss a gentle exercise programme with your doctor – it is very important to increase the exercise of each muscle gradually.

Skin and hair care

Your dry skin will improve as your thyroid hormone levels return to normal with treatment. However, it is helpful to reduce other causes of dry skin while this is happening.

Wear rubber gloves when washing up or doing other wet jobs, and avoid contact with detergents and other chemicals. Protect your skin from wind and sun. Moisturising creams may soothe itchy dryness, but it is probably better to use ones without strong perfumes that may irritate your skin. Baby oil in the bath or afterwards can also help, but be careful not to slip when getting in or out of the bath.

Conditioners may reduce some of the dryness in your hair. As the hair starts to grow again it may fall out alarmingly. This is because the new hairs are pushing the old ones out. Gradually, though, your hair will resume its previous thickness.

Summary

- The treatment of myxoedema is thyroxine.
- Thyroxine treatment should be started with small doses, which are increased gradually according to response.
- Treatment is usually for life.
- Thyroxine is simply a replacement for a natural hormone, so its only effects are those of the natural hormone. There are no side effects if the correct replacement dose is used.
- Watch your diet – eat more fibre and starchy foods and less fat and sugar.
- If you smoke, STOP.
- Ask your doctor about a gentle, carefully graduated exercise programme to tone and strengthen your muscles and improve your stamina.
- Protect your skin from damage and use a non-irritant moisturising cream.

8
Underactive Thyroid – Complications

Most people with an underactive thyroid start to feel better within days of beginning thyroxine replacement treatment and gradually continue to return to normal. This process may take several months, or occasionally years, depending on how severe the thyroid insufficiency was to start with. But a few people have problems, either with their treatment or because of their myxoedema itself.

Problems with Treatment

Undertreatment

If you are not taking enough thyroxine, your symptoms and signs of myxoedema will not resolve completely. If you still have any of your original symptoms after two months on the same dose of thyroxine, or if the symptoms disappear initially but then come back, contact your doctor. He can check you over generally and also send a blood sample to the laboratory to measure your TSH level and your free T4 or free T3.

If the TSH is still above normal or the free T4 or free T3 are low, you need a bigger dose of thyroxine. If, however, your thyroid hormone levels and TSH are normal, it may mean that your body is taking a long time to get used to normal thyroid hormone levels, or that the symptoms that are still troubling you are not actually due to myxoedema.

There is another problem with thyroid replacement treatment, though. Some people simply do not take their pills. It may seem very obvious, but if you do not take your thyroxine, it cannot cure your myxoedema. Thyroxine replacement therapy is not like a course of antibiotics – taken for a week and that's that. It is usually for the rest of your life – every day, every week, every month, every year. The occasional missed pill will not be a disaster, but a lot of missed pills will mean that you do not get the full benefit of your treatment.

Another cause of undertreatment (or overtreatment) is failure to understand the dosage of thyroxine, lack of communication or error. In Britain the pills come in 25 microgram, 50 microgram and 100 microgram strengths. A

50 micrograms (mcg)
or 0.05 milligrams (mg)

100 micrograms (mcg)
or 0.1 milligrams (mg)

50 mcg

100 mcg

150 mcg

200 mcg

Doses of thyroxine.

microgram is a thousandth of a milligram. Some doctors may write the dose down as 0.1 milligram (mg) instead of 100 micrograms (0.1 milligrams and 100 micrograms are one and the same thing). This has led some patients to inform me that they are on 1 milligram a day, whereas others assure me that they are taking 'point oh one' daily. Some people even insist that the prescribed dose was 100 milligrams daily.

It is most important that you realise what strength pills you have and that you know how many pills you should take to make up your dose. Check the bottle each time you get a new supply from the pharmacist – is it the same dose as before? The dose ranges from 25 micrograms to 300 micrograms, but the vast majority of people end up on 100 or 150 micrograms a day; 100 micrograms is two 50-microgram pills or one 100-microgram pill.

Thyroxine is a once-a-day medication and it is sensible to take it each morning when you wake up so that you do not forget it. I have met people taking it twice or even three times a day, in divided doses. It is a long-acting drug and it is not necessary to split the dose like this, although you will come to no harm if you do divide it up. If there is any confusion in your mind, the most sensible idea is to take the bottle to the doctor or hospital or pharmacist every time. It's no use just showing them one pill, without the bottle – people keep doing this to me. But have you any idea how many types of little white pills there are?

Overtreatment

We all feel slightly unwell occasionally and anyone with a busy life feels tired sometimes. But if someone is feeling slightly unwell or complains of feeling tired, and they are known to have myxoedema, it is tempting for both patient and doctor to blame the symptoms on the thyroid problem. 'Let's increase the thyroxine,' they say, 'that will improve things.' It may do, but only if the symptoms are actually due to a thyroid hormone lack.

Overtreatment, due to patient or prescriber error, is fortunately rare, but the examples above should alert you to this potential problem. Thyroid function blood tests will quickly demonstrate whether overtreatment is occurring. If the TSH is very low, the person is receiving too much thyroxine, which will be suppressing pituitary TSH release. High levels of free T4 in the blood also suggest this, although slightly raised free T4 is not uncommon in thyroxine therapy (it simply shows that the pills you are swallowing are being absorbed). A high level of free T3 – the active form – is more worrying and suggests that the thyroxine dose should be reduced.

It is very rarely necessary for anyone to take more than 300 micrograms of thyroxine daily. Resist the temptation to keep increasing the dose if you do not feel quite right. Each year I see few patients who are taking larger doses than this, who look thyrotoxic and whose thyroid function tests confirm excess thyroid hormone. It is possible to get 'hooked' on the adrenaline-like buzz of thyroid excess and it can be very difficult to reduce the dose.

You may recognise overtreatment because it causes the symptoms of thyroid overactivity (see Chapter 9). There is some evidence which suggests that overtreatment increases thinning of the bones – osteoporosis. It is therefore important to avoid excess thyroxine. However, under-treatment may cause a rise in the blood cholesterol level, increasing the risk of coronary artery disease. A careful balance, avoiding either over-replacement or under-replacement, is, therefore, best, although this is sometimes easier in theory than in practice.

Complications of Thyroid Underactivity

Heart problems

Myxoedema can damage the heart in three ways:

- By encouraging furring-up of the arteries supplying oxygen and nutrients to the heart (coronary atherosclerosis).
- By weakening the heart muscle generally.
- By causing accumulation of fluid (effusions) in the bag which surrounds the heart (pericardium). This is called pericardial effusion.

The most common heart problem found in people with myxoedema is coronary atherosclerosis and its consequences. This occurs because of the increase in cholesterol circulating in the bloodstream associated with thyroid underactivity. It can cause angina (page 171) and, rarely, a heart attack or coronary thrombosis. If the myxoedema is treated and the cholesterol level returns to normal, the furring-up of the arteries may regress, although very long-standing hard lesions in the arteries may be permanent. Always tell your doctor if you have a pain in your chest. But remember, however, that most pains in the chest are not due to heart attacks.

Weakening of the heart muscle is called cardiomyopathy. It is debatable whether this is simply due to poor circulation or previous heart attacks from coronary atherosclerosis, or whether there is a separate myxoedematous cardiomyopathy, i.e. the weakening of the heart muscle is caused directly by the myxodema. Both this and pericardial effusion can cause shortness of breath and pitting ankle swelling, i.e. the swelling pits if you prod it. See your doctor if you have either of these symptoms.

Hypothermia

People with myxoedema have a very slow rate of metabolism and therefore find it difficult to keep warm. Rarely, elderly people – usually those whose thyroid insufficiency has not been diagnosed are admitted to hospital with hypothermia. Hypothermia *(hypo* means low, *thermia* means heat) is a condition in which the person is unable to maintain their body temperature, so that they gradually cool down.

If you have an elderly relative with recently diagnosed myxoedema, be especially careful to help them keep warm in cool weather. Once the thyroid hormone levels have returned to normal, though, they will respond to cold like anyone else of their age.

Myxoedema coma

This is now a rare complication of myxoedema and, again, is most likely in older people, especially if the condition is undiagnosed, or is in the early stages of treatment.

If someone has very severe myxoedema or their condition is complicated by a major illness, the body metabolism may slow down so much that they become unconscious. They may become hypothermic as well. Myxoedema coma requires urgent treatment in hospital. Call an ambulance if you cannot wake up a myxoedematous person.

Summary

- There are few complications of myxoedema.
- Undertreatment may be due to too small a dose of thyroxine, error or failure to take the pills regularly.
- Overtreatment may be due to increasing dosage for symptoms unrelated to myxoedema, or impatience as it takes time to return to normal.
- The commonest complication is coronary atherosclerosis

and its consequences – this troubles few people and is treatable.
- Hypothermia and myxoedema coma are rare.

9

Overactive Thyroid – Symptoms

Other names for an overactive thyroid gland are hyper-thyroidism (*hyper* means high) and thyrotoxicosis. Graves' disease is the association of thyrotoxicosis, goitre and protruding eyes described by Robert Graves in 1835. The term now tends to be used for autoimmune thyrotoxicosis and I will refer to this as Graves' disease for simplicity. As in Chapter 3, symptoms are listed according to the body system to which they relate.

How common are the symptoms of thyrotoxicosis?

Symptom	Percentage of people with thyrotoxicosis who have the symptom
Nervousness	99
Increased sweating	91
Oversensitive to heat	89
Palpitations	89
Fatigue	88
Weight loss	85
Fast heart	82
Shortness of breath	75
Weakness	70
Increased appetite	65
Eye complaints	54

Swelling of legs	35
Frequent bowel action	33
Loose motions	23
Loss of appetite	9
Constipation	4
Weight gain	2

General Behaviour

Anxiety and nervousness Some people with an overactive thyroid feel as if their body is rushing out of control. You may feel as if things are going too fast for you and you would very much like them to ease up. Some people simply have a vague feeling of anxiety or inner confusion. A few people feel so anxious that they go to their doctor for tranquillisers, 'to calm my nerves, doctor'.

Mood changes You may find that you are euphoric, 'over the moon' one minute and in the depths of depression the next. You may find yourself snapping at people, irritable and knowing that you are being unreasonable but unable to stop yourself. You may be impatient. Less often, you may believe that people are messing you about and feel suspicious of offers of help. I sometimes meet people with thyrotoxicosis who refuse to believe their thyrotoxicosis needs treating. They may be angry and aggressive. They see me and their other doctors as interfering. Once they have been persuaded to accept treatment and the T3 and T4 are nearer normal they realise how much they needed help and are very grateful that their doctors persisted. On other occasions you may suddenly burst into tears over a minor problem, or apparently over nothing at all. Your family and friends may find this very difficult to cope with, and close personal relationships may suffer. These mood swings are due to the thyrotoxicosis and are called emotional lability; they will settle as the thyroid hormone levels return to normal.

Overactivity People with thyrotoxicosis can feel a compulsion to keep active, and may be completely unable to sit and rest. 'I always want to be on the go.' 'I can't bear sitting doing nothing.' 'I'm such a fidget, I just can't keep still.' You may clean around your family, or be always up and down rearranging things or tidying. At work you may fidget or want to rush decisions. You can be a little difficult to keep up with.

Talkativeness It may be your family and friends rather than you who first notice how talkative you've become. You may have so much to say, so quickly, that you cannot stop talking, and no one else can get a word in edgeways. Indeed, on one occasion, I was compelled to put a thermometer into a thyrotoxic person's mouth to keep them quiet for just long enough for me to listen to their heart.

Tiredness and exhaustion The problem with thyrotoxicosis is that, although you are bursting with ideas and want to do everything yesterday, you may not have the stamina to carry it out. You may become tired easily and start jobs, only to discover that you cannot finish them. It is easy to become frustrated. In severe thyrotoxicosis you may become completely drained with the demands of your overactive metabolism, and become exhausted. Instead of burning to rush about all the time, all you want to do is sleep, and everything seems too great an effort. This is quite a worrying symptom in someone with thyrotoxicosis: firstly, it may not be immediately obvious that you have the condition, so that it may take longer to diagnose; and secondly, it means that your body is drained of energy and you are in urgent need of help (see page 121). Your tiredness may be increased by sleep disturbance and nightmares.

Skin, hair and nails Your skin may be smooth, thin, hot, pink and moist. You may also have areas of darker skin pigment than usual. Women with thyrotoxicosis often complain of blushing very easily, the blush usually extending down the neck on to the top of the chest and lasting for some time. Your palms may be particularly red. Many of the symptoms of thyrotoxicosis mimic those of anxiety; anxiety also causes sweaty palms, but someone with thyrotoxicosis will find their hands sweaty all over. Indeed, excess sweating can be an embarrassing problem. Some people notice itching.

About one in 20 people with thyrotoxicosis develop a skin condition called pretibial or localised myxoedema. These swollen red/purple patches, fading to brown, are usually found on the shins (hence pretibial). Occasionally they occur elsewhere on the body. They are rarely troublesome and usually disappear. Some doctors use steroid treatments if they are sore or fail to settle.

Thyroid acropachy is another uncommon condition linked with thyrotoxicosis. In about one in 100 people the fingertips and nails become curved and bulbous. It looks a little unusual but is rarely a problem. Most people with thyroid acropachy have pretibial myxoedema.

Your nails may separate and accumulate dirt easily. Your hair may become very soft, fine, fly-away and difficult to control; you may find more of it in the comb or brush than usual. About one in three people with thyrotoxicosis notices hair loss.

A swollen neck Many people with thyrotoxicosis will have a goitre, i.e. a swelling of the neck. Quite often it is just an appearance of fullness in the front of the neck, but if the thyroid swelling is larger, necklaces or shirt collars may become tighter. Contrary to popular belief it is unusual for goitres to cause pressure inside the neck, and swallowing and breathing are hardly ever affected.

Heart, Circulation and Lungs

Heat intolerance If you have thyrotoxicosis, even in the

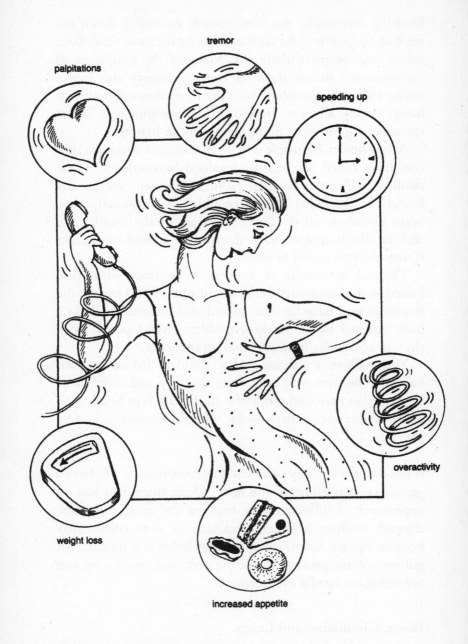

Symptoms of thyrotoxicosis.

coldest weather your overactive metabolism and vigorous circulation can make you feel hot. When everyone else is closing windows and putting on extra woollens, you are so hot you cannot bear it. You fling the bedclothes off at night, open the windows and turn the central heating down – your partner may not appreciate this at all. At work, you may still be in summer clothes while everyone else dons winter wear. You may also notice that your skin is very pink and feels hot to the touch, reflecting your vigorous circulation. Rarely, you may actually have a raised body temperature.

Increased sweating Many people with thyrotoxicosis also notice increased sweating; for example, you may find yourself sweating profusely after minor exertion. This, combined with feeling hot, may make you wonder if you have a fever.

Palpitations As the increased thyroid hormones speed up the metabolism, the heart has to beat faster. You may become aware of this as an uncomfortable feeling or fluttering in your chest, especially at night, but also when you exercise. You may feel your heart pounding fast, usually in a regular rhythm, but sometimes erratically. It is very helpful for your doctor to know whether the heart beats are evenly spaced (e.g. ******) or unevenly spaced (** * *** * * **) and, if possible, how fast your heart is beating during an episode of palpitation – try feeling your pulse (see page 161) and count the rate with your watch. Some people have intermittent palpitations – the heart starts beating fast when they have not been exercising at all. And rarely, the heart may go so fast that you feel faint or dizzy – your doctor needs to know about this.

Shortness of breath This may be a part of your general lack of stamina – many people with thyrotoxicosis become puffed on hills, going upstairs or carrying heavy shopping. If you feel very breathless, especially while you are having palpitations, you should contact your doctor straightaway – he may need to give you some treatment to steady your heart. Severe thyrotoxicosis may weaken the chest muscles and cause shortness of breath.

Digestive System

Increased appetite You may start to feel hungry all the time. Second and even third helpings disappear quickly. You can start eating large snacks or have midnight feasts. Your friends look on enviously as you tuck into a huge helping of spaghetti bolognese – 'I don't know how you can eat all that and still stay slim.' But a few people, usually those with a very overactive thyroid, lose their appetite.

Weight loss If your thyroid is overactive, your metabolism speeds up and you start to burn up first of all your fat stores and then, if the condition is not treated, your other body tissues. Even though your appetite increases, you lose weight, the weight loss sometimes being rapid. Occasionally, the increase in appetite is so great that people actually gain a little weight, but this is unusual.

Vomiting This is an uncommon symptom of thyrotoxicosis. It may presage thyroid storm (see pages 100 and 121).

Diarrhoea Different people mean different things when they talk about diarrhoea. Most people with thyrotoxicosis need to open their bowels more often than usual, but the motions are normally formed. Alternatively, you may also have loose or runny motions. Sometimes the motions smell bad and float. These pale, greasy stools are due to impaired absorption of fat.

Muscles and Bones

Shakiness Tremor or shakiness of the hands is a classical feature of thyrotoxicosis. It is present all the time, but is particularly obvious when you hold your hands out-stretched. An artist with thyrotoxicosis found that drawing in fine detail was difficult because of this shaking. If you have to handle precision instruments you may have difficulties. The tremor is probably due to the increased sensitivity to adrenaline – the fright, flight and fight hormone – and is just like the shaking we all get when we are frightened or anxious.

Muscle weakness Although your thyrotoxicosis drives you to start a lot of energetic tasks, you may find that your muscles are too weak to achieve them. This weakness is often especially severe in the thighs and sometimes the upper arms. You may have difficulty walking upstairs, getting up after squatting or getting out of the bath. Because it affects the muscles closest to the trunk, it is called proximal myopathy. Sometimes your muscles may seem strong enough to start the job but tire easily. Your muscles may become thinner too – the medical term is muscle wasting.

Bones Prolonged thyrotoxicosis can also thin your bones, causing osteoporosis. This may produce aches and pains, particularly in the back.

Sex and Periods

Irregular or absent periods Medical students tend to assume that thyroid overactivity is linked with frequent, heavy periods. In fact, the opposite is the case. Your periods may stop altogether, especially if you have lost a lot of weight. Someone who usually has regular periods may find them occurring at longer or shorter intervals, with little blood loss or just spotting.

Sexual drive or libido In men this may be reduced. Some women with thyrotoxicosis have an increased sexual drive. You may find intercourse tiring because of muscle weakness.

Fertility Abnormal or absent periods reduce women's fertility. Thyrotoxic men may have a low sperm count with reduced motility.

Male breast enlargement or gynaecomastia Most thyrotoxic men develop some excess breast tissue. All men make some of the female sex hormone, oestrogen. In thyrotoxicosis oestrogen levels rise. This also explains the reduced libido and sperm problems. The gynaecomastia is rarely very obvious and settles on treatment of the thyrotoxicosis.

Eyes

Most people are aware of the link between fullness of the eyes and the thyroid gland. This condition, although very closely linked to thyrotoxicosis, is separate and is therefore considered in a separate chapter (pages 133–139).

Summary

- An overactive thyroid gland is also called hyperthyroidism or thyrotoxicosis. Graves' disease is the combination of thyrotoxicosis, goitre and protruding eyes.
- General symptoms of thyroid overactivity include anxiety, nervousness, overactivity, talkativeness and tiredness.
- You may also feel heart palpitations, increased sweating and shortness of breath.

- Weight loss, despite increased appetite, and diarrhoea can occur.
- Other symptoms include shakiness, muscle weakness, menstrual and sexual problems.
- These symptoms resolve with treatment.

10

Overactive Thyroid – What the Doctor Looks For

Your Story

As with an underactive thyroid – indeed, with all medical problems – it helps your doctor if you can list the symptoms which are troubling you most and if you can tell him as much as you can about them. How long have you had them? Have you ever had them before? What makes them better or worse? And so on. Remember that no one has all the symptoms on the list and some people do not notice any of them.

Previous medical history

Remember all your previous major illnesses and operations. Have you ever had a thyroid problem before? Do you have diabetes, Addison's disease or pernicious anaemia?

Family history

Do you have a family history of thyroid disease or of other autoimmune disorders (see page 46)?

Your job and lifestyle

What are your work and home commitments? Are you coping with the demands of your overactive thyroid gland and your work? Is a young family wearing you out when you are already tired and weak with your thyrotoxicosis?

Eating, drinking and smoking The caffeine in coffee and tea may add to your shakiness and speed up your heart rate if you drink too much. Alcohol causes flushing because it increases the circulation to your skin, and alcoholic drinks may add to your heat intolerance. And if you smoke, be honest about the number of cigarettes you get through a day. Then start working out how you are going to stop.

Drugs and medicines. Allergies I have already discussed the drugs which may interfere with the older thyroid function tests (see page 38). But some other drugs may mask your symptoms of thyrotoxicosis – the beta blockers (atenolol, metoprolol, propranolol) for example. Some people with thyrotoxicosis may be given tranquillisers before it becomes obvious that their problem is not their nerves but their thyroid gland; these too may modify some of your symptoms. The dose of some drugs may need increasing until T3 and T4 return to normal (see page 123).

You must tell your doctor if you are allergic to any medication.

Examination – Looking for Signs

General behaviour and appearance People with severe thyrotoxicosis may be so overactive that the air about them seems to quiver – I call this an agitated aura. With these patients the interview can sometimes be quite a problem for the doctor, particularly if the patient is very overactive and talkative. It is hard to get a word in edgeways and examining someone who cannot keep still can be challenging. One of the lessons I have learned is that the patient who gets the doctor feeling all worked up is probably thyrotoxic.

If you are thyrotoxic you are likely to be slim, with loose-fitting clothes. You may be wearing lightweight garments, even in cold weather, and will almost always have taken off your outer layers of clothing in the warmth of the hospital or health centre.

Hands Your handshake will usually be very warm and your skin may feel rather moist. Your rings may be loose. The palm of your hand may be red (palmar erythema). Your nails may separate from the nail bed at the tips, which makes them break easily and it can also be hard to clean dirt out from underneath. This condition is called onycholysis or Plummer's nails. You may have thyroid acropachy. If you hold your hands outstretched in front of you, your fine tremor will be obvious — especially if the doctor lays a piece of paper on top of your hands.

Skin and hair Your skin is likely to be smooth, warm and pink and you may have the 'thyroid flush' from your face down on to your chest. This can linger blotchily on your chest for some time after the flush has ebbed from your face. (Some women blush like this normally.)

Some people with thyrotoxicosis develop pretibial myx-oedema (see page 73). You may have small patches of puffy thickening in other areas and some people with thyro-toxicosis develop a thickening of the skin on the jawline. Your hair may be thin and fine.

If you have an autoimmune thyroid disorder (see page 46) you may develop areas of pigment loss on the skin or in the hair. These white patches are called vitiligo in the skin and leucotrichia in the hair. They are simply a signal of autoimmune trouble and are not due to thyroid hormone problems. The white areas of skin burn easily and should be

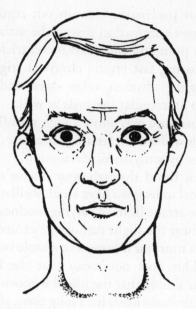

A person with thyrotoxicosis.

covered with sun block in hot sunshine. They can be camouflaged with makeup if their appearance troubles you.

Neck Many people with thyrotoxicosis have a goitre (see Chapter 17). Your doctor will feel your thyroid to see if the goitre is smooth or lumpy. Because the blood supply to the thyroid has increased, your doctor may be able to hear the turbulent blood flow as a whooshing noise through his stethoscope. This noise is called a thyroid bruit.

Heart, circulation and lungs Your pulse will be fast (tachycardia) unless you are on beta-blocker medication. Your heart rhythm may be irregular – called atrial fibrillation because the problem is due to an irregular quivering of the atria or upper heart chambers. Normally, the area of nervous tissue in the heart that controls the beating of the heart – the heart pacemaker – sends out regular electrical stimuli that trigger contraction first of the atria and then of the lower, main pumping chambers or ventricles. But if the atria start producing fast erratic electrical triggers of their own, this irregular rhythm takes over and makes the ventricles pump at irregular intervals as well.

Your blood pressure may show a high systolic (pumping) pressure and a low diastolic (resting) pressure. This reflects your vigorous or hyperdynamic circulation.

Your heart, as heard through your doctor's stethoscope, will sound normal unless you have atrial fibrillation, in which case there will be erratic beats of varying loudness. Sometimes the doctor can hear the slight turbulence caused by vigorous blood flow and a murmur is present in systole (when the heart is pumping). This does not mean that the heart is malfunctioning, but simply that the blood is moving fast. If you have had severe thyrotoxicosis for a long time, your heart may have become weakened, and you may have developed swollen ankles with pitting oedema (see pages 16–17).

There are unlikely to be any abnormalities in the lungs unless you smoke.

Abdomen Occasionally, people with an overactive thyroid develop a swollen liver which can be felt under the ribs on the right of your abdomen. This will return to normal with treatment.

Eyes Your eyes may show some of the changes described in Chapter 16.

Nervous system Your tendon reflexes are likely to be very brisk – indeed, the doctor may be able to elicit them simply by tapping your knees with his finger.

Muscles If you have lost a great deal of weight, your muscles may be thin and generally weak. This particularly applies to the thighs. If your doctor asks you to squat down and then stand up without using your hands to help, you may not have the strength to do so.

Case History of Thyrotoxicosis

Maria Stow is a 55-year-old art teacher in a college of further education. This is her case history, as written down by her doctor.

Patient complains

- 'I'm losing weight.'
- 'I feel the heat very much.'
- 'My hands are shaky.'

History of presenting complaint

Mrs Stow has always had difficulty losing weight, but over the past two months has lost 2 stone (28 pounds or 12.7 kg), despite eating more than usual on holiday in Spain. Her appetite has increased and she wakes up hungry in the night and raids the fridge. She usually enjoys hot weather, but on this holiday was unable to tolerate it. She has turned the central heating down at home, and has had arguments with her husband as she keeps throwing the covers off the bed at night because she feels so hot and sweaty. They are now sleeping in separate beds. She teaches drawing and has been unable to draw fine lines because of increasing shakiness of her hands over this period.

On direct questioning, Mrs Stow has also noted increasing fullness in her neck, although is unsure when this started, and sometimes experiences fast regular palpitations, especially on exercise. She used to open her bowels about every two days but now does so once or twice a day. The motions are normal in colour and consistency.

Previous medical history

- Fractured left leg ski-ing 1968.
- Pernicious anaemia 1977.

Social and family history

- Married, husband an engineer.
- Three children, one married, two still at home.
- Lives in a four-bedroomed house.
- Non-smoker.
- Drinks about two bottles of wine a week.
- Diet mainly vegetarian, but eats dairy produce and fish.

Family history

- Her mother had diet-treated diabetes, while her maternal grandmother had goitre.

Drugs

- Vitamin B12 injections for pernicious anaemia.
- Occasional paracetamol for headache or backache.
- Temazepam in the past month for sleep.

Allergies

- None known.

Direct questions

- *Cardiovascular and respiratory system:*
  Short of breath on exertion.

No cough or sputum.
No chest pain.
Palpitations as above.
No ankle swelling.

- *Gastro-intestinal system:*
Increased appetite.
No nausea or vomiting.
No indigestion or abdominal pain.

- *Genito-urinary system:*
No pain or bleeding on urination.
No increased frequency of urination.
Menopause three years ago.
No post-menopausal bleeding.

- *Nervous system:*
Occasional headaches.
No fits, faints or falls.
Vision normal.
Hearing normal.
No paraesthesiae (tingling).

- *Musculoskeletal system:*
Muscles slightly weaker generally than usual.
Occasional backache for 10 years at least.
Occasional pain in left leg since fracture.
No joint pains.

- *Endocrine system:*
No thirst, polydipsia (drinking a lot) or polyuria (passing
large volumes of urine).

- No postural dizziness.

On examination

- Height 5 foot 7 inches (1.7 metres).
- Weight 7 stone 10 pounds (49 kg) (ideal weight 8 stone
4lb to 10 stone 7lb – 53–67 kg).
- Overactive, talkative, grey-haired, blue-eyed woman.
- Vitiligo on the arms and trunk.

- Warm, moist skin.
- Flushed.
- No anaemia.
- Fine tremor of outstretched hands.
- Bilateral exophthalmos (bulging eyes); lid lag and lower lid retraction; full eye movements; normal conjunctivae.
- Bilateral smooth thyroid enlargement; soft bruit over right thyroid lobe.

Cardiovascular system

- Pulse 100 beats/minute, regular rhythm.
- Blood pressure 170/60.
- No venous engorgement.
- Heart not enlarged.
- Heart sounds normal; systolic flow murmur.
- Normal peripheral pulses.
- No ankle oedema.

Respiratory system

- Trachea central.
- Expansion normal.
- Percussion note and breath sounds normal.

Abdomen

- No masses or organ enlargement felt.

Nervous system

- Cranial nerves normal, including hearing and vision.
- Retinae normal.
- Power, tone, coordination and sensation normal in all limbs.
- Reflexes present, equal, very brisk.

Diagnosis

* Thyrotoxicosis.
* Treated pernicious anaemia.

The next section of the case notes would consider confirmatory investigations and health checks, followed by treatment and general health advice. These are considered in Chapters 11 and 13. The causes behind Mrs Stow's thyrotoxicosis can be found on page 94.

Summary

* Signs of thyrotoxicosis include agitation, talkativeness, overactivity, slimness and hand tremor.
* The skin may be warm, pink and sweaty.
* There is often thyroid swelling or goitre.
* The heart rate is usually rapid and the tendon reflexes are brisk.

11

Overactive Thyroid – Tests

Thyroid Function Tests

The measurement of T3 and T4 has already been discussed (see Chapter 5).

In thyrotoxicosis the free T3 and free T4 will be raised. The total T3 and total T4 will also be raised, but it is important to check that you are not taking any pills which will raise the carrier protein levels and give a false impression of thyrotoxicosis.

As the T3 and T4 levels in your blood rise, so your TSH produced by your pituitary will fall, and eventually its release will be switched off completely. These very low levels of TSH cannot be detected by some of the older TSH assays; however, most laboratories are using a highly sensitive assay system which can detect these tiny quantities of TSH. The TSH levels mentioned throughout this book assume that a highly sensitive assay has been used.

These are Mrs Stow's results, with normal range in brackets.

- Free T4 48 picomol/1 (9–24 picomol/1).
- Free T3 12 picomol/1 (2.5–5.3 picomol/1).
- TSH under 0.05 milliunit/1 (0.3–5.0 milliunit/1).

Extremely rarely, the pituitary gland develops a tumour

which overproduces TSH, which in turn forces the thyroid to overproduce T3 and T4. In this case the T3, T4 and TSH levels would all be raised.

The TRH test

As in hypothyroidism (see pages 40–41), this test is used in borderline cases. If you have an overactive thyroid, the pituitary will release very little TSH in response to stimulation by an injection of thyrotrophin releasing hormone (TRH). This flat response confirms the diagnosis.

Thyroid antibodies

Just as in hypothyroidism, the body may make antibodies to the thyroid gland – anti-microsomal and anti-thyroglobulin antibodies (see page 46). The other antibodies involved in the development of thyrotoxicosis cannot be measured routinely (see pages 94–98).

Thyroid scan

If you have one or more lumps in your thyroid, and in some other instances, your doctor will request an imaging scan of the thyroid. There are several ways of doing this.

An ultrasound thyroid scan is a simple way of looking at the consistency of the thyroid. It is similar to the scans which assess your baby in pregnancy. Some jelly is put on your throat and a probe moved over the skin. You may find the pressure uncomfortable briefly. Ultrasound can usually distinguish cysts from solid lumps and a multinodular goitre from the smooth one of Graves' disease (see Chapter 9).

The radioactive iodine scan (this is not the same as having radioactive iodine treatment for your overactive thyroid) involves an injection of a tiny dose of radioactive contrast into a vein. Sometimes other isotopes are used. The iodine is taken up most avidly by the parts of the thyroid that are most active in producing thyroid hormones. In this way the scan may show up a single overactive nodule which could then be removed surgically to cure the condition.

Other Tests

Blood count

The white blood count may be lower than normal in some people with an untreated thyrotoxicosis. Pernicious anaemia may co-exist with either hypothyroidism or thyrotoxicosis (as in Mrs Stow) (see page 152).

Liver function tests

While the thyroid is overactive the liver may temporarily malfunction. This liver damage can be detected by transiently raised blood levels of enzymes (special chemicals) normally retained in liver cells.

Blood proteins are also made in the liver, so their levels may fall if the liver is not working properly.

Blood calcium concentration

Up to one in five people with thyrotoxicosis have a raised blood calcium concentration (see page 122), the causes of which are complex.

Blood glucose concentration

Diabetes should be excluded in everyone with a thyroid disorder by measuring the blood glucose concentration. People with diabetes have high blood glucose levels.

Electrocardiogram

This is needed to check the heart rhythm, especially in atrial fibrillation.

Summary

- In thyrotoxicosis blood concentrations of free T4 and free T3 are high.
- TSH levels are very low.

12

Overactive Thyroid – Causes

The causes of thyrotoxicosis are shown in the table below. While most doctors agree that autoimmunity is responsible for most thyroid disorders in the United Kingdom, whether overactivity or underactivity, there is considerable debate as to the precise sequence of events in both conditions. The situation is particularly complicated in thyrotoxicosis.

Causes of thyrotoxicosis

Autoimmune (Graves' disease) 80 per cent
Toxic multinodular goitre 15 per cent
Toxic nodule 2 per cent
Thyroxine overtreatment
Thyroiditis
Excess iodine intake
Excess TSH (very rare)
Ovarian tumour (very, very rare)

Graves' Disease

For many years scientists have known that people with thyrotoxicosis have chemicals in their blood which cause the thyroid gland to produce excessive thyroid hormones. Further work has identified an antibody which can bind to the areas on the surface of thyroid cells usually reserved for thyroid stimulating hormone from the pituitary – the TSH receptors. Therefore this TSH receptor-stimulating (TSHRS) antibody stimulates the thyroid to overwork, causing thyrotoxicosis. This form of thyroid overactivity can occur in a previously normal-sized thyroid gland or in one that has become enlarged, for example in an area of iodine deficiency.

A receptor is a place on the surface of a cell where a chemical can link with that cell. It is rather like a keyhole waiting for a key. Several keys may fit into the keyhole, but usually only one turns the switch to make something happen. In this case the keyhole or TSH receptor is designed for the TSH key, but the TSHRS antibody key not only fits the keyhole but turns the switch as well.

But why does the body make the TSHRS antibody? One

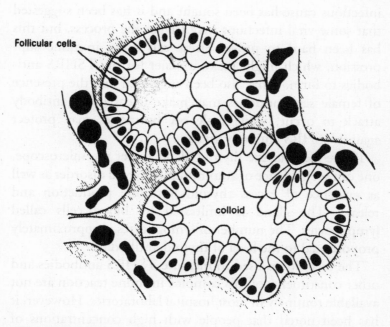

Follicular cells

colloid

Thyroid follicles as seen under the microscope in thyrotoxicosis. Note the depleted colloid stores.

theory is that the thyroid cells themselves are the cause of their own downfall. They may have slightly abnormal TSH receptors which trigger the production of the TSHRS antibody, which then comes back and stimulates the over-production of thyroid hormones.

Another theory is (as with myxoedema) lack of protection against self-attack; people with a tendency to autoimmune disorders inherit a flaw in their surveillance mechanism. Consider the immune mechanism as a security force in a large manufacturing plant; in the case of this particular flaw, either the security guards are asleep and fail to detect the pro-duction of the TSHRS antibody, the potential saboteur, or they are alert but carry guns without bullets and cannot shoot the saboteur down before it overstimulates the thyroid.

There is much discussion about what triggers the formation of TSHRS antibodies or begins their attack. An infectious cause has been sought and it has been suggested that some viral infections may trigger the process, but this has been hard to prove. Stress can cause immune sup-pression, which might make it easier for the TSHRS anti-bodies to form. It has also been suggested that the presence of female sex hormones may make it easier for antibody attack to occur, while male sex hormones may protect against TSHRS antibody attack.

If one looks at the thyroid gland under the microscope, one can see evidence of autoimmune thyroid disorder as well as evidence of excess thyroid hormone production and release. The gland is infiltrated by blood cells called lymphocytes. The number of lymphocytes is approximately proportional to the level of thyroid antibodies.

The techniques used to measure TSHRS antibodies and other constituents of this complex immune reaction are not available routinely in most hospital laboratories. However, it has been noted that people with high concentrations of thyroid stimulating antibodies often have high concen-trations of anti-microsomal antibodies, and this can be used as a clue to what is happening. Other blocking antibodies, which stop the TSH receptor from working, may also be found in people with thyrotoxicosis – which is why you may spontaneously become myxoedematous. This tendency for thyroid conditions to swing from one extreme – thyrotoxicosis – to the other – myxoedema – makes it very difficult to predict what will happen to someone with thyroid trouble, and makes it hard to assess the effects of treatment.

Toxic solitary thyroid nodule and toxic multinodular goitre

In these conditions one or more parts of the thyroid gland start producing thyroid hormones on their own. These areas which become swollen or lumpy (i.e. nodular) no longer follow the control system via the pituitary gland and TSH release but 'do their own thing'. These autonomously functioning thyroid nodules (AFTNs in some American literature) can occur alone in normal thyroid glands or may be found in multinodular goitres (see page 140). If you have an AFTN within a normal thyroid gland, it overproduces thyroid hormone and causes thyrotoxicosis. It is as if a small group of workers in the thyroid factory decides to work overtime, even though their product is surplus to requirements. This suppresses pituitary TSH levels which switches off thyroid hormone production in the normal part of your thyroid.

If you have AFTN(s) in a multinodular goitre you may have normal thyroid hormone levels or be thyrotoxic. The blood thyroid hormone levels depend on the size of the AFTN(s) and how much iodine is available in your diet. If the AFTN is bigger than 2.5 cm (1 inch) you are more likely to become thyrotoxic.

The proportion of cases of thyroid overactivity due to these causes varies considerably depending on the amount of iodine in the local diet. The rate is higher in iodine-deficient areas. Among patients with thyrotoxicosis, studies have found 3 to 11 per cent due to toxic solitary nodule and 5 to 21 per cent due to toxic multinodular goitre.

The cause of AFTNs is not entirely clear. Some of them may stimulate their own TSH receptors, causing over-production of thyroid hormones. It does seem that the problem lies within the nodule itself. The earliest sign may be reduced TSH levels. In this situation the T3 may be high (and detected) before a rise in T4 occurs – T3 thyro-toxicosis. T3 thyrotoxicosis can also occur with other unusual thyroid lesions. It may be some time before the person feels any symptoms of thyrotoxicosis.

Thyroid nodules and multinodular goitres are discussed in more detail in Chapter 17.

Thyroxine Treatment

People with myxoedema may sometimes take too much

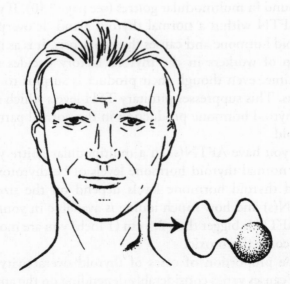

Thyroid nodule.

thyroxine, either because of an error or because they do not realise that the dose must be controlled carefully (see pages 56–58). Alternatively, if someone with normal thyroid function takes thyroxine they may well develop the signs and symptoms of thyrotoxicosis, especially if they take it in large doses; this may occur if someone with borderline myxoedema is given inappropriate thyroxine. Some doctors also use thyroxine to shrink thyroid nodules, although this is unlikely to cause thyrotoxicosis as most doctors monitor thyroid function regularly in this situation.

People occasionally take thyroxine as a slimming aid. It must be emphasised here that the only use for thyroxine indicated in the *British National Formulary* is the treatment of thyroid disease.

Thyroiditis

Viral infections can cause thyroid inflammation, which may produce a temporary increase in the release of thyroid hormones from the damaged cells. The diagnosis of thyroiditis can be confirmed by a thyroid scan, which will show low activity in the thyroid gland because of the inflammation. This differentiates it from the more chronic condition of thyrotoxicosis, in which there is a high uptake reflecting the overactivity of the gland and its vigorous blood supply.

Excess Iodine

Too much iodine, for example in an attempt to correct dietary iodine deficiency, can switch on thyrotoxicosis in someone with an iodine-deficient goitre. This is called the Jod-Basedow phenomenon. Nowadays, perhaps the commonest cause of thyrotoxicosis due to excess iodine intake is the heart drug amiodarone. This can also cause myxoedema. Thyrotoxicosis is more likely if the person has previously had a low iodine diet. Arniodarone also has other effects in the thyroid and perhaps the pituitary.

TSH Overproduction

Overproduction of TSH by the pituitary gland is a very rare cause of thyrotoxicosis indeed.

Hyperemesis gravidarum (excessive vomiting in pregnancy)

Occasionally women with hyperemesis gravidarum may develop temporary thyrotoxicosis due to the stimulating effect of the pregnancy hormone human chorionic gonadotrophin (hCG) on the thyroid. Once the vomiting has settled with treatment the thyrotoxicosis resolves. Treatment with antithyroid drugs is not needed unless the patient has underlying thyrotoxicosis from another cause.

Summary

- Thyroid overactivity is usually due to disturbances of the person's own immune system – autoimmunity. This causes Graves' disease.
- Thyroid nodules may produce excess thyroid hormone.
- Excess iodine can cause thyrotoxicosis in someone with an iodine-deficient goitre.
- Viral thyroiditis can cause temporary thyroid overactivity.
- Thyroxine overtreatment and TSH overproduction are rare causes of thyrotoxicosis.

13

Overactive Thyroid – Treatment

There are three ways of treating an overactive thyroid. Everyone will receive medication to start with. For many people this is sufficient to calm the thyroid and, over months or years, maintain normal function. However, tablets offer only a temporary solution in most cases. It is possible to remove some of the overactive gland surgically. The third treatment is radioactive iodine.

Deciding on the best treatment for you is something for you and your doctor to consider, so what follows is a general guide only.

The decision as to which treatment to use depends on many factors. These include your preferences, age, sex, whether you are pregnant or planning pregnancy, whether you are breast feeding, the cause of your thyrotoxicosis (e.g. Graves' disease or multinodular goitre, see pages 94–98), the severity of your thyrotoxicosis, whether it is your first episode of thyrotoxicosis or not, the size of your goitre, previous side effects of anti-thyroid treatment, the presence of other illnesses', local facilities and the preferences and experiences of your doctor.

In medicine, if there are many ways of treating a condition it usually means that there is no single best treatment but a variety of options. For example, a survey of UK practice a few years ago found that there are over 100 different ways of giving radioiodine treatment for thyrotoxicosis! This can be difficult for you as a patient, particularly if you see different doctors for your thyroid – they may all give different advice. A consensus statement for good practice in the management of thryoid disease was published in the *British Medical Journal* in 1996 (see page 169). The information given in this book is generally in accordance with the consensus statement, but you may find it helpful to read the paper for yourself. Further studies have increased our understanding of the management of thyrotoxicosis (see pages 168–170).

Anti-Thyroid Medication

Indications for anti-thyroid medication

Nearly everyone with newly diagnosed thyrotoxicosis from any cause is treated with anti-thyroid drugs initially to stop the T3 and T4 levels rising further and prevent worsening of the condition. The aim then is to return the thyroid function to normal. The exception is thyrotoxicosis due to thyroiditis, in which damage to the thyroid cells causes leakage of thyroid hormone into the bloodstream. Anti-thyroid drugs will not help as the problem is leakage, not overproduction.

Long-term options are:

• Continue on anti-thyroid drugs for six months to two years.
• Continue on anti-thyroid drugs until your thyroid function is normal and then have radioiodine or surgery.

The course of anti-thyroid treatment

A large dose of anti-thyroid drug is used to start with. After that there are two patterns of anti-thyroid drug treatment – to tailor the anti-thyroid drug according to thyroid function tests, aiming for the smallest effective dose; or to continue to give a big dose to 'block' the thyroid and add thyroxine (block and replace). Both have their advocates. Block and replace treatment is simpler and requires fewer medical checks than tailored treatment. However, people using block and replace have to swallow more pills, and may have a greater risk of side effects. Block and replace should not be used in pregnancy.

If you have Graves' disease and this is your first episode of thyrotoxicosis, many doctors would give you a prolonged course of anti-thyroid drugs. This is because there is a chance of long-term remission. One can rarely say that someone with Graves' thyrotoxicosis is 'cured' as the condition may reappear many years later. It is difficult to predict who is likely to gain long-term remission on anti-thyroid drugs.

A group in Birmingham, England, studied the outcome of treatment of patients with Grave's thyrotoxicosis. In those only receiving tablets, tailored doses of anti-thyroid drugs (mainly carbimazole) were given for 18 months. Six months after stopping the tablets only 40 per cent of the women, and just 20 per cent of the men still had normal thyroid function. The rest had recurrent thyrotoxicosis. The age at diagnosis also influenced the success of anti-thyroid tablet treatment. Treatment was successful (for the first six months) in 33 per cent of those under 40 years old as compared with 48 per cent of those of 40 years old or over. Even if treatment appears successful for the first six months, thyrotoxicosis can recur in later years.

Initial remission may be more likely on a block and replace treatment (70 per cent) than on tailored treatment (40 per cent). With tailored treatment, the longer the treatment, the greater the chance of long-term remission. Two years after treatment ends, approximately 40 per cent of people after a six-month tailored course of treatment are free from thyrotoxicosis, and about 60 per cent after a two-year course. Two-year remission rates for courses of block and replace treatment are about 50 per cent whether the treatment last six months or a year. Fifty to 60 per cent of patients on any form of tablet treatment will have had another episode of thyrotoxicosis within five years. Most of the relapses occur within a year and most of the remaining recurrences happen within five years. So, if your thyrotoxicosis has not recurred within five years of stopping tablet treatment, then it is unlikely to do so.

So, ultimately, there appears to be little difference in the relapse rate following tailored treatment or block and replace. By five years, at least half the people on either form of treatment will have relapsed.

Many endocrinologists give everyone a high dose of antithyroid drug initially and then choose the treatment pattern that seems appropriate for that patient, taking into account their preferences, their ability to swallow pills and what has happened to their thyroid function. One way of deciding is based on the thyroid hormone changes on treatment. If it proves easy to tailor the dose and you feel well and are happy with the treatment, then you carry on with tailored treatment for two years. If the thyroid hormone levels fall too low or go up and down, making you feel ill, then you could use block and replace for six months. Proponents of block and replace would say that one should use this anyway to prevent major ups and downs in thyroid function.

If you have severe thyrotoxicosis or a big goitre, the chance of any remission is small. You are also more likely to relapse if you have high levels of anti-microsomal thyroid antibodies (see page 42). If this is your second episode of thyrotoxicosis, the chance of remission of thyrotoxicosis with anti-thyroid drugs is about 10 per cent. The same applies if you do not take your tablets regularly as prescribed!

Some people opt to continue a small dose of anti-thyroid drugs for ever. They have usually had several episodes of Graves' thyrotoxicosis or have a toxic nodular goitre and may not wish to explore other options. It appears safe and convenient.

There are three forms of medication which reduce thyroid hormone production – carbimazole, propylthiouracil and Lugol's iodine solution. Propranolol relieves symptoms of thyroid overactivity and may also have a direct effect on thyroid hormones.

Carbimazole

Carbimazole blocks the incorporation of iodine into thyroid hormone precursors and inhibits further steps in the chemical pathways in the thyroid. It also influences the autoimmune process and reduces antibody attack on the thyroid gland. In the body it is converted to the active drug, methimazole, and it is this form that is used in North America and elsewhere instead of carbimazole.

Carbimazole pills come in 5 mg or 20 mg strength each. They are prescribed as a large starting dose, to achieve a rapid effect in controlling the thyroid, followed by a gradually decreasing dose according to response until a maintenance dose is reached. The maximum starting dose is 60 mg a day, but this is rarely needed and many doctors start with 30 mg a day. The response to carbimazole is very variable. You may have near normal T4 levels in a month, or it may take as long as six months on a high dose of carbimazole before your thyroid responds fully to treatment. The dose is then reduced over several months according to response, until a maintenance dose is reached – usually 5 to 15 mg daily. There is some discussion as to whether the dose should be taken all together once a day or divided up. The pills work equally well in most people either way. However, in severe thyrotoxicosis the pills should be taken every six hours, because of rapid metabolism. Once the thyroid hormone levels are stable you can be seen by your doctor about every three months.

Block and replace treatment aims to suppress the immune reaction causing the thyrotoxicosis. It starts with 40 to

60 mg carbimazole daily as above. Once the T4 is normal (or low), 40 mg carbimazole is taken once a day with thyroxine 100 to 150 micrograms. Thyroid hormone levels are checked in about a month if they are normal, then you will be seen every three to four months. Block and replace is usually continued for six months.

Once you have finished your course of treatment, someone (either your general practitioner or your endocrinologist) should check you regularly for five years. One option is to have formal thyroid function tests every six months, but to ask you to attend for a blood test straightaway if you notice any symptoms of thyrotoxicosis. Practice varies. I believe that you should then have a thyroid hormone check annually for ever, but other doctors would say that this results in a lot of blood tests to identify a few people with thyroid problems.

Some people will develop spontaneous myxoedema in the years after their thyrotoxicosis has settled. Estimates of this happening range from 2 to 20 per cent. Ultimate myxoedema is more likely if you have microsomal antibodies (see page 42).

Contraindications and warnings A contraindication is an indication that a given sort of treatment should not be used. In the case of carbimazole, the first contraindication is a previous adverse reaction to carbimazole. Carbimazole should not be taken long term by people with very large goitres or those who have goitres pressing on the trachea (or windpipe) – this is because the drug can cause the thyroid to swell even further. Caution is needed in people with liver disease. The manufacturers advise not to breast feed while taking carbimazole.

Side effects Two to five per cent of people on carbimazole have side effects. The most important, which affects fewer than one in 100 people taking carbimazole, is that of lowering the white blood cell count. The white blood cells help to fight infection, the granulocytes by eating bacteria and the lymphocytes by making antibodies (see page 42). If carbimazole reduces your granulocyte count, it can render you liable to infections, particularly sore throats (although it should be remembered that some people have a low white blood cell count, due to thyrotoxicosis itself, before they start treatment – see page 92).

Red blood cells may fall, causing anaemia. Platelets, tiny particles which help the blood clot, may fall, causing easy bruising or bleeding. If you develop a sore throat, mouth ulcers, fever, infection, anaemia, easy bruising or bleeding while you are taking carbimazole, stop the drug straightaway. Go to your doctor or a hospital emergency department for a blood count within 24 hours. This reaction is rare but is most likely to happen in the early months of treatment. It is usually temporary. The blood count returns to normal once the carbimazole has been stopped.

Skin rashes – for example, itchy red spots – sometimes occur with carbimazole treatment and settle once treatment is stopped. Sometimes they are so mild that it is not necessary to discontinue treatment. Some hair loss may also occur. Other side effects are nausea, loss of taste, headaches, aching joints, swollen lymph glands and fever, tingling and numbness, jaundice, diarrhoea, swelling, hair loss, rhinitis and conjunctivitis.

Propylthiouracil

Like carbimazole, propylthiouracil inhibits the incorporation of iodine into thyroid hormones. It also blocks conversion of T4 to T3 in some tissues.

Propylthiouracil is usually made in 50 mg pills, the usual initial dose being 450 mg, either all taken at once or divided through the day. The dose will then be reduced, according to response, to a maintenance dose of 300 mg a day or less.

Contraindications Breast-feeding mothers should ensure their baby's thyroid function is checked if taking 150 mg or more a day. Propylthiouracil should be used with caution in people with poor kidney function. It should not be used in people with very large goitres or those who have goitres pressing on the trachea.

Side effects The tablets taste bitter so should be swallowed quickly. Side effects occur in about three out of every 100 people who take the drug. They are the same as those of carbimazole, so it is important that you read the warning about low white cell count (page 106) carefully. A low white count is slightly rarer in people taking propylthiouracil than those on carbimazole.

Lugol's iodine solution

This is only a temporary treatment – it is used before thyroid surgery and occasionally in very severe thyrotoxicosis. Lugol's iodine solution is a drink containing iodine and potassium iodide dissolved in water, the dose being 0.1 to 0.3 ml three times a day.

Contraindications Iodine therapy should be used with great caution in pregnant women and should not be given to breast-feeding mothers – it can cause goitres in their babies.

Side effects Some people are allergic to iodine – you must tell your doctor if you are. Allergic reactions to iodine can include symptoms of a cold, headaches, watery or red eyes, sore throat, bronchitis or skin rashes. Iodine is only given for a short course of treatment – long-term side effects include myxoedema, depression and impotence.

Propranolol

This is a beta-blocker – it blocks the effects of adrenaline (the fright, flight and fight hormone) on the heart, blood vessels, lungs and elsewhere. This means that propranolol calms the feeling of nervousness experienced by so many people with thyrotoxicosis, slows the heart rate down and steadies the overactivity. It may also limit the conversion of T4 into the active thyroid hormone T3.

Propranolol pills come in several strengths – 10 mg, 40 mg, 80 mg and 160 mg. This makes it especially important for you to know what dose you are taking. The usual dose in thyroid overactivity is 20 mg three times a day. Some people need more, however. The maximum dose of propranolol is 320 mg in 24 hours, but this much is rarely used in thyrotoxicosis and the more usual dosage range is 10–40 mg three to four times a day (a total of 40–160 mg in 24 hours). The dose will then be tailed off gradually as you start to feel better as a result of other anti-thyroid treatment.

Sometimes, the doctor may start you on propranolol to relieve your symptoms while awaiting the result of diagnostic thyroid blood tests. Because propranolol improves your symptoms and signs of thyroid overactivity, you and your doctor can no longer rely on a clinical assessment as a guide to how overactive your thyroid gland is. You will thus have to rely mainly on the results of blood tests from now on.

Contraindications People with asthma or a wheezy chest should never be given propranolol, as it may precipitate a severe or even fatal attack. It reduces circulation in the blood vessels to the arms and legs, and so should not be given to people with problems in these arteries. It also reduces the pumping power of the heart – harmless in people with normal hearts. If you have heart failure it may make it worse – except, in most instances, in thyrotoxicosis when it is used with caution, and may improve the heart problem by calming the heart rate.

Side effects A slow pulse, heart failure, wheezing, reduced circulation in arms and legs, aching muscles, lack of energy, sleep disturbance, bad dreams and gastrointestinal disturbances. People with insulin-treated diabetes may lose their warning of hypoglycaemia (a low blood glucose) if they take propranolol.

Radioiodine Treatment

This means swallowing a small dose of radioactive iodine so that it will be taken up by the thyroid and will gradually inactivate some or all of the thyroid hormone producing cells, depending on the dose given. The affected cells are gradually destroyed. In most cases the aim is to reduce thyroid hormone production to normal levels. In some people the aim is to stop thyroid hormone production completely. Note that radioiodine treatment cannot be guaranteed to cure thyrotoxicosis and it may cause thyroid underactivity. The radioactive isotope used is iodine 131. There are published guidelines for the use of radioiodine in the management of thyrotoxicosis (Royal College of Physicians, 1995, see page 169).

Indications

Toxic nodular goitre (see page 97) Thyrotoxicosis due to toxic nodular goitre rarely remains in remission on anti-thyroid drug treatment only.

A toxic nodule (i.e. one which is causing thyrotoxicosis) (see page 97) should take up the radioiodine, leaving the rest of the thyroid untouched. This is the simplest treatment for toxic thyroid nodules. A fine needle aspirate should be taken as these nodules may very rarely be cancerous (page 143).

Graves' disease (see page 94) In this condition many doctors would try a course of anti-thyroid drugs first, although some would give radioiodine initially, especially in elderly people. In the USA radioiodine is often used to treat thyrotoxicosis. If anti-thyroid drugs do not control the thyrotoxicosis reliably or if you are unable to take them (because of side effects, for example), then radioiodine is an option. If the thyrotoxicosis recurs, then a second course of anti-thyroid drugs is unlikely to produce a long-term remission. Again, radioiodine is indicated.

The Birmingham group studied radioiodine treatment for thyroid over activity from several causes. After six months, one dose of radioiodine was less likely to resolve thyrotoxicosis in men (68 per cent) than women (77 per cent). Younger patients, those with larger goitres, and those with severe thyroid over activity were more likely to need a second dose of radioiodine. There are many ways of adjusting the radioiodine dose, but calculated doses of radioiodine, tailored to the individual, do not seem to have any benefit over fixed doses in the ultimate cure rate, or thyroid under activity rate.

Contraindications or cautions

Pregnant women or breast-feeding women should not be given radioiodine (see page 129). If you are planning pregnancy, wait at least four months after radioiodine before stopping contraception.

It has been suggested that thyroid eye disease may be worsened by radioiodine treatment. Although this may not, in fact, be the case, there is still debate and it would seem sensible to avoid radioiodine in thyrotoxic people with active thyroid eye disease unless no other treatment is appropriate or works. Steroid treatment can be given to protect the eyes in this situation.

Radioiodine should be given with caution to people with very large goitres, as these may become inflamed and swell after treatment. However, eventually the goitres usually get smaller.

People with severe uncontrolled thyrotoxicosis may develop thyroid crisis (see page 121) after radioiodine. Antithyroid drugs should be used to control overactivity if at all possible.

Allergy to iodine.

Problems protecting other people from radiation. These can usually be resolved – for example, if someone has urinary incontinence a catheter can be inserted.

If your thyrotoxicosis follows amiodarone therapy, your thyroid will be packed with iodine and radioiodine treatment may not work very well.

What does radioiodine treatment involve?

Radioactive iodine is given as a drink like water or as a capsule. It is tasteless. It has to be given under supervision of a doctor with a certificate in the Administration of Radioactive Substances from the national Advisory Committee (ARSAC). It must also be given in a 'controlled area' – a room complying with the ionising radiation regulations. This may mean seeing another doctor, for example a radiotherapist, in another department for your radioiodine treatment. The regulations and the need to go somewhere else can make radioiodine treatment seem more dramatic than it really is. It is usually a very straightforward treatment.

After you have swallowed the radioactive iodine, most of it will be taken up by your thyroid gland and the remainder will leave your body in the urine in about two days. You will be given instructions about special precautions after the radioiodine. These will vary depending on the dose you have received. The aim is to reduce unnecessary radiation to other people, especially young children or pregnant women. Everyone will be asked to avoid close contact with other people for at least one day, and avoid close contact with children and pregnant women for at least a fortnight. If you have a bigger dose of radioiodine, you will be asked to stay off work and avoid public transport for one or two days. Most people are treated as out-patients – admission is only needed if you are given more than 800 milliBecquerels (MBq) of radioiodine, if you have uncontrolled severe thyrotoxicosis or if you are unwell for some other reason.

How much radioiodine?

There is a wide variation in the dose of radioiodine given by different doctors. Some may do tests to tailor the dose for you beforehand, although others may feel that this is unnecessary. The dosage range is from 200 to 800 MBq; 800 MBq is the dose which usually stops the thyroid working. The usual dose to normalise thyroid function is about 300 to 550 MBq. You can have another dose two months later, if necessary.

What about anti-thyroid drugs?

An overactive thyroid gland takes up radioiodine avidly. So radioiodine works best in untreated thyrotoxicosis. Some doctors give you propranolol to relieve the symptoms and calm the heart rate and use radioiodine straightaway. However, there is a risk of releasing a lot of thyroid hormone into the circulation as the radioactivity destroys thyroid cells. This can cause you to feel very unwell (very thyrotoxic) or, rarely, precipitate thyroid crisis.

Most doctors would first control the thyrotoxicosis with anti-thyroid drugs and stop them at least four days before radioiodine treatment. Block and replace treatment should be stopped a month beforehand. Anti-thyroid drugs can be restarted, if necessary, three days after treatment. Most people will not need further anti-thyroid drugs. You can continue your propranolol throughout, if necessary.

Follow up

Always report any symptoms of thyroid overactivity or underactivity to your doctor straightaway. Do not wait for your next appointment. Have a thyroid hormone check about six weeks after treatment and again six weeks after that. The intervals thereafter depend on your thyroid hormone state. Eventually you will be in a stable thyroid state. Everyone who has ever had radioiodine treatment should have annual thyroid function tests for life.

Questions which worry people

People advised to have radioiodine treatment usually worry about their future children and about any risk of cancer to themselves.

The guidelines state: 'Forty years of experience in using radioiodine has shown no effect on the utero development and subsequent health of children of patients who have had this treatment, beyond the normal incidence of congenital disease.'

People are always concerned that radiation, even in the tiny doses used in radioiodine treatment, may cause cancer in the future. Several large studies have examined this issue. One study looked at over 7,000 Birmingham people treated with radioiodine for thyrotoxicosis. Overall, people treated with radioiodine had a significantly lower risk of cancer than the rest of the population. There were significantly fewer deaths from cancer in the radioiodine-treated people compared with the expected mortality in the population in general. This is very reassuring. The only individual cancers which were more likely in patients treated with radioiodine were those of the thyroid and small bowel, and only 15 people in the entire group had one of these cancers. An American study looked at the influence of thyrotoxicosis itself upon cancer mortality and found that there is a small increase in the likelihood of thyroid cancer even in patients who had not had radioiodine. It should be emphasized that thyroid cancer is uncommon, and responds well to treatment. In the American study of thyrotoxic patients treated in a variety of ways and followed for an average of 21 years, only 29 out of 33,748 patients died from thyroid cancer (0.09 per cent as compared with 0.03 per cent in the general American population) (see Chapter 17).

Problems with radioIodine treatment

Myxoedema Most people given radioiodine treatment will develop an under active thyroid at some point. The timing depends on several factors, but by about 20 to 30 years after treatment nearly everyone given radioiodine will need thyroxine replacement. This is why some doctors deliberately aim to make the thyroid under active straightaway – so that there is less need for monitoring over the years while awaiting the development of myxoedema. The Birmingham group found that 61 per cent of people given 370 MBq of radioiodine were on thyroxine replacement one year later. The development of thyroid under activity depends on the dose of radioiodine given. However, lower doses of radioiodine were not very effective in treating the thyrotoxicosis. Thyroid under activity was more likely to develop in people treated with radioiodine for Grave's thyrotoxicosis than in those with toxic nodular goitre. High levels of thyroid antibodies also pre-disposed to myxoedema.

Thyrotoxicosis and thyroid crisis The dose of radioiodine may be insufficient to cure the thyroid overactivity and, as described above, there may be transient worsening of the thyrotoxicosis due to excessive hormone release (see page 121).

Inflammation of the thyroid Occasionally, the reaction

caused by the radioiodine inside the thyroid causes inflammation, and the gland may become swollen and sore, although this thyroiditis is usually temporary. The salivary glands occasionally become inflamed too.

Lumpy thyroid In later years, the thyroid gland may develop nodules after radioiodine treatment.

Thyroid Surgery

This is indicated for big goitres, especially lumpy ones; the rare ones which press on the trachea or other neck structures; for people under 45 years old who keep having recurrences of

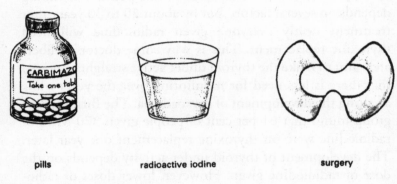

| pills | radioactive iodine | surgery |

Treatment of thyrotoxicosis.

thyrotoxicosis; and for young people who cannot take anti-thyroid pills for any reason. Some younger women will opt for surgical treatment because a medium-sized goitre worries them or because they do not wish to take anti-thyroid pills. Planned pregnancy may be another reason.

As with all treatments of thyrotoxicosis there are many different opinions. Some doctors, especially surgeons, believe that all young people with an overactive thyroid should be offered surgical treatment. Others rarely use surgery. This variation in attitudes may reflect local expertise in thyroid surgery. Like all surgical procedures, someone who specialises in thyroid surgery may be expected to obtain better results than someone who rarely operates on the thyroid. There are so many areas of specialisation in surgery that one cannot expect every district to have a specialist in thyroid surgery.

Preparation for operation

It is dangerous for anyone with thyrotoxicosis to have any operation unless the thyroid hormone levels have been returned to normal by treatment, otherwise surgery can precipitate a thyroid crisis. Before the operation you need treatment with carbimazole or propylthiouracil and propranolol, probably for about two months, then for the last fortnight most surgeons would advise Lugol's Solution. This makes the thyroid easier to handle at operation, as well as reducing thyroid hormone levels.

Most surgeons would also insist on a detailed examination of your voice box to check the vocal cords. This is carried out by an ear, nose and throat specialist (otorhinolaryngologist), using a mirror to look down the back of your throat, and is done because about three people in 100 have a weak vocal cord without realising it, and the operation carries a very small risk of damaging the nerves which supply the vocal cords.

The operation itself – a partial thyroidectomy – requires a general anaesthetic, so the anaesthetist will check you before the operation. The operation then consists of the removal of about two-thirds of both lobes of the thyroid gland.

Winding down behind the thyroid is the recurrent laryngeal nerve – the nerve that goes to the vocal cords – which, as we have seen, can occasionally be damaged at operation. The other problem is that deep within the thyroid gland lie the four parathyroid glands which are responsible for organising calcium balance. The surgeon will search carefully for them so that they are left intact.

Problems of thyroid surgery

Myxoedema About two out of 25 people who have thyroid surgery develop myxoedema (thyroid underactivity) in the years after surgery, those with high levels of thyroid microsomal antibodies being particularly at risk. Some surgeons remove most of the thyroid gland, aiming to produce myxoedema, and prescribe thyroxine routinely after operation. As with large doses of radioiodine, this can be useful for people who have had very troublesome ups and downs of thyroid hormone levels over months or years of anti-thyroid treatment.

Recurrent thyrotoxicosis This is uncommon but can occur and occasionally nodules develop in the thyroid remnant.

Bleeding Rarely, a small blood vessel may bleed into the neck. This can create a painful blood clot, causing pressure on the windpipe, so it may have to be drained quickly.

Hoarse voice Sometimes (in about three in 100 cases), the recurrent laryngeal nerve is bruised at operation or becomes a little inflamed during the healing reaction after surgery. In this case the vocal cords do not work properly and you may become hoarse for a few weeks or several months. But it is very rare for the vocal cord to be permanently damaged.

Low blood calcium concentration If the parathyroid glands have been bruised at operation, or their blood supply has been inadvertently reduced, they may temporarily stop working. This can lead to the blood calcium level falling dramatically and can cause you to become weak, with cramping spasms in your hands. The cure is calcium pills or injections, followed by vitamin D pills. This situation usually resolves completely, as the parathyroid glands settle down after the operation. If it does not, you will need long-term calcium supplements.

Wound problems After the operation you will be left with a scar following a wrinkle line across your neck ask the surgeon to show you where it will be before the operation. It usually fades until it is virtually indistinguishable from a wrinkle. Very rarely, the scar becomes lumpy.

Other problems All anaesthetics carry a very small risk of problems, and all operations carry small risks of damage to other local structures, of infection and of thrombosis.

Discuss all of the above, and any other worries you may have, with your surgeon. But you should always remember that the risk of problems is very small and the vast majority of people who have thyroid surgery have no complications.

Table 13.1 Treatment options for thyrotoxicosis

Problem	Treatment which is often advised
Newly diagnosed thyrotoxicosis	Anti-thyroid medication (e.g. carbimazole) initially
Children/young people/ pregnant women	Anti-thyroid medication Thyroid surgery
Graves' disease	Anti-thyroid medication Radioiodine Thyroid surgery
Graves' disease (20 to 40 years old, high T4 levels, men)	Radioiodine
Large goitres	Thyroid surgery Radioiodine (unless risk of compression of underlying structures)

Goitres compressing underlying structures	Thyroid surgery
Multi-nodular goitres (lumpy)	Thyroid surgery Radioiodine
Overactive thyroid nodule	Thyroid surgery Radioiodine

There are many different ways of treating thyrotoxicosis. Discuss the treatment options for your thyrotoxicosis with your own doctor and decide together which option will suit you best.

Summary

- The treatment of thyrotoxicosis is complex. Different patients need different treatments and different doctors use different treatment regimens.
- Because thyrotoxicosis is a fluctuating condition, and because people's responses to treatment vary, the effects of treatment can be difficult to predict.
- Pills – carbimazole or propylthiouracil – suppress the production of thyroid hormone. Propranolol relieves the symptoms of thyrotoxicosis.
- Most people are treated with these pills at first.
- Radioactive iodine destroys some of the overactive thyroid tissue.
- Surgery – partial thyroidectomy – which removes about two-thirds of the thyroid is another option, especially for large goitres.
- Radioiodine and surgery may cause permanent myxoedema.
- All treatments may be followed by recurrent thyrotoxicosis.
- A person with an overactive thyroid needs regular medical follow up for life.

14

Overactive Thyroid – Complications

Exhausted Thyrotoxicosis

Sometimes people with thyrotoxicosis are not overactive, talkative or nervous. Instead they lie in bed, exhausted, quiet, depressed and too weak to do much to look after themselves or their family. It is as if the constant stress on their body from the excess thyroid hormones has 'burnt them out'. Older people with thyrotoxicosis are more likely to be apathetic or even depressed. This is a potentially dangerous situation and requires treatment in hospital with carbimazole or propylthiouracil, and fluids and nutrients, if necessary.

Thyroid Crisis

In a person with severe, untreated thyrotoxicosis or with inadequately treated thyrotoxicosis, a physical shock (such as an infection, an operation or an accident), or radioiodine treatment can cause a thyroid crisis. This is when the excess thyroid hormones cause a high fever, a very fast pulse and collapse, sometimes with vomiting, diarrhoea, dehydration or jaundice. It is the body's response to the thyroid hormones rather than to the actual concentrations of T3 and T4 that is important. Another name for this condition is thyroid storm.

This uncommon and dangerous condition requires

immediate hospital treatment to cool and rehydrate the person and control the thyrotoxicosis with large doses of carbimazole, Lugol's iodine solution and propranolol.

High Blood Calcium Level

About one in five people with thyrotoxicosis has a raised blood calcium level. If the level is very high it can cause vomiting, thirst and frequent urination, passing large volumes of urine (polyuria). The mechanism for the rise in blood calcium is complex, but the problem will usually settle as the T3 and T4 levels fall. Another reason for thirst and polyuria is diabetes.

Heart Problems

Most people with thyrotoxicosis have a faster heart rate than normal. About 10–15 per cent have an irregular heart rhythm called atrial fibrillation. This may be present all the time, especially in elderly people, in whom it may be the first sign of overactive thyroid. It can occur intermittently. You may feel very uncomfortable for a while, with an erratic pounding in your chest and occasionally feeling faint or short of breath.

The heart rate and rhythm usually return to normal as the thyroid overactivity settles. Sometimes the atrial fibrillation may persist (particularly in older people). In this situation, especially if you have high blood pressure, or other heart problems such as disease of the coronary arteries or heart valves, you should be considered for anticoagulant (blood-thinning) treatment with drugs like warfarin. This is to prevent clots forming in the heart and causing a stroke.

Thyrotoxicosis may cause heart failure, again mainly in older people. Heart failure means that the heart does not pump as vigorously as it should and the person may develop swollen ankles or shortness of breath due to fluid accumulation. Thyroid overactivity alone can make the heart pump less strongly than usual, but most thyrotoxic people who develop heart failure also have high blood pressure or atrial fibrillation or coronary artery disease. Treatment is usually very effective. It involves anti-thyroid measures (see page 102), diuretics (water-losing medication) and digoxin (a drug which calms atrial fibrillation and helps the heart to pump more strongly).

Tests your doctor may do include a heart tracing or electrocardiogram (sometimes recording the heart rhythm over 24 hours on a small recorder worn on a belt) and echocardiogram in which an image of the heart is produced by placing an ultrasound probe on the chest in different positions.

Bones

Thyrotoxicosis can cause loss of bone density (osteoporosis) and an increased likelihood of fractures, particularly in women, and especially after the menopause. Even after the thyrotoxicosis is treated there may some risk of osteoporosis so it is sensible to keep this under review with your doctor. Make sure you have a well-balanced diet with a good calcium intake. Your doctor may advise calcium supplements. After the menopause, sex hormone replacement therapy may also help to protect your bones. Regular exercise (appropriate for your general state of health) can help keep your bones strong.

Effects of Thyrotoxicosis on Drugs

Thyrotoxicosis increases your body's metabolic rate (the rate at which chemicals are processed in the body). It also increases the clearance of many chemicals from the body. This means that T3 and T4 themselves disappear more rapidly from the body, as do other hormones. This is why you are asked to take anti-thyroid drugs in divided doses during the day in acute thyrotoxicosis (i.e. a dose of carbimazole of 30 mg a day is taken as 10 mg three times a day). This rapid clearance may affect many drugs – for example, the blood levels achieved by the same dose of digoxin for heart problems may be halved by thyrotoxicosis. The effect of this may be that your usual medication is no longer effective. Occasionally the dose needs to be increased – then reduced again as the T3 and T4 return to normal. Discuss this with your doctor.

Summary

- Serious complications of thyrotoxicosis – exhaustion and thyroid storm – are rare.
- High blood calcium levels occur in one in five people with thyrotoxicosis, most of whom have no symptoms of calcium excess.
- Heart problems are usually transient, but heart failure may occur in elderly people.
- Thyrotoxicosis may cause thinning of the bones (osteoporosis).
- Check whether you need to adjust your medication while you are thyrotoxic.

15
Pregnancy

Thyroid problems do not stop you from having a baby. Among 1,000 births in one large maternity unit in one year, two were in women with thyrotoxicosis and nine in women with myxoedema. Untreated thyroid disorders (particularly myxoedema) may make it harder for women to become pregnant (see page 24). However, it is possible to become pregnant with mild untreated myxoedema or thyrotoxicosis. The outcome of pregnancy for both mother and baby may be better if the thyroid disorder is treated as soon as it is discovered, although problems are uncommon. If you know you have a thyroid condition, it is better to use contraception until the thyroid hormone levels are normal on treatment. Then stop the contraception. Thyroid disease may improve temporarily during pregnancy. It may also occur for the first time during or immediately after pregnancy.

The areas considered in this chapter are the changes of normal pregnancy, myxoedema, thyrotoxicosis and thyroid swelling. Where relevant, the effects on both the mother and the baby will be considered.

The management of thyroid disease in pregnancy is a specialist field in which knowledge is increasing all the time. If you are planning pregnancy or actually pregnant, it is essential that you see an endocrinologist as soon as possible, to help you to normalise your thyroid function before pregnancy to ensure that it remains normal during and after pregnancy. The endocrinologist will work closely with the obstetrician (doctor for pregnancy) and the paediatrician (children's doctor) or neonatologist (doctor for newborn babies). Because knowledge is changing and endocrinologists' views vary, it is essential that you discuss your particular thyroid problem and its treatment with your specialist. What I have said in this book may not apply to you.

Changes in Pregnancy

In pregnancy the way you feel and look changes. The symptoms and signs of normal pregnancy can mimic those of thyroid disorders, making it difficult to know if what you are experiencing is due to your thyroid or the pregnancy itself. Cessation of periods, nausea, sweating, heat intolerance, palpitations and shakiness occur in most pregnant women, and in thyrotoxicosis. Weight gain, fluid retention, puffiness, lethargy, constipation and carpal tunnel syndrome (see page 19) could be signs of myxoedema – or pregnancy.

In most women the thyroid gland swells as pregnancy progresses. This is a normal response to the increased iodine demands of pregnancy. The thyroid is generally swollen and feels soft. It gradually goes down in the year after pregnancy unless you have a low iodine diet (rare in the UK, where food is supplemented with iodine).

During pregnancy thyroid hormone levels alter. Free hormone assays should be used to assess thyroid status in pregnancy. Total T3 and T4 levels are difficult to interpret. They are greatly elevated because rising oestrogen causes a large rise in thyroxine binding globulin levels during pregnancy. Different studies vary in their assessment of what happens to free hormone levels in pregnancy. This may be partly due to the variable effects of other pregnancy changes on the assays. By the third trimester free T4 and free T3 fall. TSH drops in the first two trimesters and rises in the third.

Myxoedema in Pregnancy

Mother

If you have myxoedema and are planning pregnancy, ensure that you are taking exactly the right amount of thyroxine to keep your TSH normal and your T4 within the normal range or just above normal. It may be helpful to check your T3 as well. Most pregnant women who were on an adequate dose of thyroxine before pregnancy do not need to adjust their dose as pregnancy progresses. Some endocrinologists routinely increase the dose of thyroxine during pregnancy, but this practice seems to be becoming less common. T3 and T4 cross the placental barrier, but this is unlikely to cause problems for your baby.

If you discover that you are myxoedematous during pregnancy, start thyroxine promptly. Your endocrinologist will probably check your thyroid hormone levels every two to four weeks until they have returned to as close to normal as possible.

There is some debate as to how often pregnant women with adequately treated myxoedema should have thyroid hormone tests. The usual recommendation is in each trimester, but some doctors check them every month and others just at the third trimester.

Pregnancy is one cause of transient myxoedema – see page 131.

Baby

In untreated maternal myxoedema there is an increased likelihood of early miscarriage, congenital malformations, premature delivery reduced intelligence quotient, or stillbirth. It should be remembered that these events do occur in women who do not have thyroid problems (more than one in 10 of all pregnant women miscarry in the first trimester).

You can breast feed while on thyroxine as too little crosses into the breast milk to have a clinical effect on the baby. However, if the baby has a blood test it may show slight changes in the thyroid hormone levels.

Thyrotoxicosis in Pregnancy

Mother

Established thyrotoxicosis If you have established thyrotoxicosis it is best to plan your pregnancy and conceive once the thyroid function is normal. In most cases this can be achieved with anti-thyroid drugs. Most endocrinologists believe that the T4 should be within the normal range but some feel that it should be slightly raised so that the foetus receives the minimum amount of anti-thyroid drugs. The TSH should be normal or just below normal. (The TSH may take weeks or months to rise back to normal on treatment after prolonged overactivity.)

Endocrinologists use both carbimazole and propylthiouracil during pregnancy. However, some doctors feel that propylthiouracil is best because it may be less likely to cross the placental barrier and reach the baby. Recent reviews have suggested that placental transfer is similar with both drugs. Propylthiouracil also impedes conversion from T4 to T3 in the tissues, so the thyrotoxicosis may come under control more rapidly.

There have been rare reports of a scalp defect called aplasia cutis in babies of mothers on anti-thyroid drugs but this association is now thought to be unlikely.

The aim of drug treatment is to give the smallest dose which achieves normal thyroid hormone levels (but there is debate as to what these are in pregnancy, see page 126). There are reservations about the use of propranolol in late pregnancy as it may cause intrauterine growth delay, slow the baby's heart or drop the newborn baby's blood glucose level. Thyroid function should be monitored throughout pregnancy. How often you are checked varies – some endocrinologists see pregnant women with thyrotoxicosis every month, but others differ. Failure to control the thyrotoxicosis increases the risk of the complications of thyrotoxicosis (see Chapter 14), and blood pressure problems (preeclampsia).

Some women prefer to have definitive treatment for their thyrotoxicosis before becoming pregnant. This would usually be a partial thyroidectomy, removing sufficient thyroid tissue to attempt to ensure no recurrence of over-activity. This aims to leave you with normal thyroid function, but you may need thyroxine replacement, in which case your pregnancy is managed as in myxoedema. You should also have your calcium level checked at the start of pregnancy to make sure it is normal. Surgical removal of part of the thyroid can be performed during pregnancy (after the first trimester) but this is very rarely necessary.

Radioiodine treatment has been used in women of child-bearing age, but it is vital to ensure that you are not pregnant at the time. Once the foetus is 12 weeks old, the radioiodine could be taken up by its thryoid. The baby's thyroid would then be destroyed, causing myxoedema. Therefore, radio-iodine is never used in the treatment of thyrotoxicosis in pregnancy and no tests using radioiodine should be done.

New thyrotoxicosis in pregnancy The symptoms and signs of thyrotoxicosis may be particularly difficult to distinguish from those of normal pregnancy. However, if you are losing weight despite eating well and you are not troubled by vomiting, you should consider thyrotoxicosis.

The signs of thyroid eye disease are not normal in pregnancy and should lead to an immediate check of thyroid function.

Hyperemesis gravidarum or excessive vomiting in pregnancy may be associated with thyrotoxicosis. (See page 100).

Up to 70 per cent of women with hyperemesis gravidarum have raised thyroid hormone levels because the pregnancy hormone, human chorionic gonadotrophin (hCG), behaves like TSH to stimulate the thyroid. The thyroid hormone levels usually settle without anti-thyroid treatment. The hyperemesis itself can be treated by an obstetrician with fluid rehydration and anti-emetic medication, or a course of steroids. Rarely, an abnormal type of pregnancy called a hydatidaform mole can cause hyperemesis and raised thyroid hormone levels. This can be detected by ultrasound scans.

Occasionally, Graves' disease becomes obvious as hyperemesis gravidarum. Thyrotoxicosis persists, even after the vomiting has settled, and is likely to be associated with positive thyroid antibodies.

Baby

There is an increased risk of miscarriage, preterm labour, and stillbirth in women with untreated or incompletely treated thyrotoxicosis. Women with autoimmune thyrotoxicosis (or Graves' disease, see page 94) – the commonest type of overactivity – may have a thyrotoxic baby. This is very rare but occurs when the thyroid stimulating antibodies which cause your thyroid overactivity cross the placenta and do the same in the foetus. As the antibodies are cleared from the baby's body after birth, the thyrotoxicosis settles. A thyrotoxic foetus or newborn baby has a fast heart beat and may have a goitre.

Some endocrinologists suggest that finding high levels of thyroid stimulating antibodies in the mother early in the third trimester may predict an increased likelihood of foetal thyrotoxicosis. However, this test is not done routinely. Rarely, sufficient anti-thyroid drug crosses the placenta to cause foetal myxoedema. This may also be associated with a goitre.

Every newborn baby of every woman who has (or has had) thyrotoxicosis should have his or her thyroid function checked.

Both carbimazole and propylthiouracil can be found in breast milk, propylthiouracil in smaller amounts. However, in most women the quantities are not considered sufficient to cause problems for the baby. However, the manufacturers state that women on anti-thyroid medication should not breast feed.

Post-Partum Thyroiditis

Up to 17 per cent of women develop transient thyroid problems after birth (post-partum). This is usually due to inflammation of the thyroid (thyroiditis) in women. A family history of thyroid disease and the development of thyroid microsomal antibodies (pages 46–47) makes post-partum thyroiditis more likely.

In the first phase, two to four months post-partum, the inflamed thyroid tissue releases T3 and T4 into the circulation. About four to eight months post-partum you may become myxoedematous. As the onset is insidious you may confuse the symptoms with the tiredness of looking after a new baby – 'just being a bit run down'. The myxoedema may also be mistaken for post-natal depression.

About one in four women with post-partum thyroiditis will need continuing thyroxine treatment but, in the rest, thyroxine can be stopped three to six months after starting treatment. Thyroid hormone levels should be checked four to six weeks later and annually thereafter as one in two of these women will ultimately develop myxoedema. If you have had post-partum thyroiditis in one pregnancy you may have it again in further pregnancies.

Goitre and Thyroid Nodules in Pregnancy

Most pregnant women have a goitre (see page 140). The rare goitres which are painful and/or are not smooth and soft should be managed as in non-pregnant women (see Chapter 17), although radioactive iodine scans must not be used in pregnancy. The same applies to thyroid nodules.

Summary

- Most women with treated myxoedema or thyrotoxicosis are healthy through pregnancy and have healthy babies.
- Myxoedema and thyrotoxicosis may reduce your ability to conceive, but pregnancy may occur.
- Both myxoedema and thyrotoxicosis should be controlled before trying to conceive.
- Untreated thyroid disease carries health risks for the mother in pregnancy.
- In untreated myxoedema or thyrotoxicosis there is a risk of foetal loss or other foetal abnormalities.
- In general, the aim of treatment is to keep the thyroid hormone levels within the normal range with as small a dose of medication as possible.
- Thyroiditis can cause transient thyrotoxicosis and then transient myxoedema post-partum. Ultimately one in two of these women will have myxoedema.
- Thyroxine, carbimazole and propylthiouracil do cross the placenta but rarely cause problems for the foetus. They also cross into breast milk but rarely in significant amounts.
- Newborn babies of women who are, or who have ever been, thyrotoxic should have their thyroid function checked, as should babies of women with myxoedema.

16
Thyroid Eye Disease

People with thyrotoxicosis due to Graves' disease often have prominent eyes or puffy eyelids. This condition is called Graves' ophthalmopathy. X-ray studies have shown that virtually everyone with Graves' disease has some changes in their eye tissues on very detailed examination. However, only 30 to 45 per cent of those with Graves' disease will have visible changes and in many this will just be bright eyes or puffy eyelids. Only 5 per cent will have severe eye problems. Thyroid overactivity itself can make the eyes look staring by stimulating the muscles which lift the eyelids. The person looks startled. This effect settles as the thyroid hormone levels return to normal, but the eye disorder itself runs its own course which may, or may not, follow the thyroid hormone changes. Thus it is possible to have thyroid-related eye problems with normal, low or high thyroid hormone levels. Some people may develop eye changes over two years before there is any change in thyroid hormone production; in others eye problems become obvious years after disordered thyroid function. However, in most cases the thyroid overactivity and the ophthalmopathy occur together. The eye changes usually get worse over three to six months. They may then stay much the same for months before gradually improving.

Symptoms and Signs

The eyes may be watery and sore or gritty. They may be

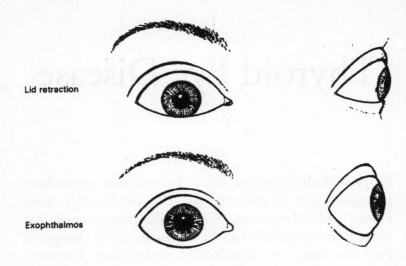

Lid retraction

Exophthalmos

Thyroid eye disorders.

slightly sticky in the morning. With severe eye problems they can become very sore. You may notice that they seem very bright and that they are bloodshot. Your vision may become blurred. You, or more often your friends or family, may notice that your eyes have become staring. Gradually the eyes may start to protrude and you may discover that you have double vision. Specific signs that your doctor will look out for are:

- *Bright eyes* Because of excess tear production or reduced drainage of tears, the eyes are a little watery and appear to gleam.
- *Blue* eyes People with autoimmune disorders are often, but not always, blue-eyed and develop grey hair early.
- *Red eyes* The white of the eye, or conjunctiva, may become bloodshot as the eye condition progresses. In severe cases the redness may be marked and permanent, and there may be swelling of the conjunctiva, giving it a wrinkled

appearance. The medical term for this is chemosis.

- *Puffy eyelids* This is especially prominent in myxoedema without other signs of thyroid eye disease. However, it often occurs in association with other eye problems, with fullness below the eyes, causing very obvious bags under the eyes, and of the upper eyelid. The lids may be a little red, especially if you have been rubbing your eyes because they feel gritty.

- *Lid lag* Your doctor may ask you to look at his finger and to follow it upwards and then down in a big sweep. He is looking for a momentary slightly jerky lag of the upper eyelid as it follows the eyeball down. Normally the eyelid moves downward smoothly with the rest of the eye.

- *Lid retraction* This is what causes the staring appearance. The upper eyelid develops slight spasm which lifts it up, exposing the white of the eye above the coloured iris which lies under the invisible cornea through which we see. Normally the eyelids cover the top and bottom edge of the iris.

- *Exophthalmos* This must be the most misspelt word in the medical vocabulary. It means sticking-out eyes, and another name for it is proptosis. To start with the eyes do not protrude very much, nor do they always protrude to the same extent. Sometimes just one eye may be affected and the doctor has to exclude other causes of eye trouble.

   The protrusion is due to oedema (fluid accumulation) in the tissues behind the eyes. The first sign may be apparent retraction of the lower eyelid, exposing the white of the eye below the iris. This is not true lid retraction, but rather the eye being pushed forwards. If the eye continues to protrude the eyelids may no longer meet over it. This means that the conjunctiva, or even the cornea, can get dry or damaged at night. This is rare.

- *Double vision* The excess fluid behind the eye can enter the muscles which move the eye. As they become swollen they do not work so well. There are separate strap-like muscles to move the eye up and down and from side to side, and if just one muscle does not work properly you will see double because the eyes cannot then be aligned properly. Looking up is often the most difficult movement.

The failure of eye muscle function is called ophthalmoplegia, and the double vision it causes is called diplopia.

- *Congestion* In severe cases, pressure builds up behind the eye, the conjunctiva becomes red and swollen because the blood vessels draining the eye are being squeezed, and the cornea may be ulcerated because the eyelids cannot close. As the pressure increases it presses on the optic nerve, which takes the visual signals from the eye to the brain for interpretation. This can cause visual loss. However, such severe damage is very uncommon nowadays.

Diagnosis and Assessment

Your doctor will obviously take a full story and examine you carefully. Your eyes will be checked in detail – what they look like, how well they move and whether they protrude. The protrusion can be measured with a device called an exophthalmometer – a small frame with mirrors that is placed beside your eyes while your visual acuity will be checked with a reading chart or an eye chart on the wall.

The doctor will also look at the back of the inside of the eye – the retina – with a magnifying torch called an ophthalmoscope. Sometimes eye drops are needed to dilate the pupil (the black part in the centre of the eye) to get a clear view of the retina; these drops may make your vision blurred for a while, but it will return to normal once they wear off. You may be referred to an ophthalmologist or eye specialist.

Obviously your doctor will check your thyroid function, and he may request scans or X-rays of your eyes or skull.

Treatment

Most people need no treatment for their eyes. The problem may worsen for a few months, level off and then very gradually improve. It can be frustrating waiting for it to settle, particularly if you are sensitive about your appearance, but the eye changes usually settle. If your eyes are dry or gritty, artificial tears (hypromellose drops) may be comforting.

It is important to keep the thyroid hormone levels normal. High thyroid hormone levels worsen the eye appearance by increasing the stare, and low levels may cause puffiness around the eyes and elsewhere. These changes may amplify those of ophthalmopathy. It is also my impression that people with ophthalmopathy who become severely myxoedematous may have a worsening of their eye problem during this time.

Severe eye changes are uncommon but can cause a lot of distress, which is why I have included this section in this book, although it will not be relevant to most of my readers. Distress is often worsened if you do not understand what is going on at each stage of treatment.

Glare is a common problem in people with thyroid eye disease. Using yellow/orange tinted glasses can reduce this by cutting out the blue part of the spectrum responsible for glare. Often just a pale tint can make the eyes more comfortable.

In severe ophthalmopathy, where the eye protrudes so much that there is a risk of corneal ulceration, large doses of steroid hormones such as prednisolone may reduce the swelling and inflammation. They are not normally used long term as prolonged high dose steroid treatment can cause weight gain, high blood pressure, diabetes, thin bones and thin skin. Occasionally cyclosporin is given. Artificial tears are used to lubricate the eye. At night gentle tape is used to close the eyelids.

Some people need surgery to decompress the orbit by removing some of the bone forming chamber in which the eye sits. Sometimes the surgeon removes some of the swollen fatty tissue behind the eye. Decompression can be done at any stage, but surgery to correct double vision is not normally done until the eye has been stable for some months. Most double vision can be treated with prisms or an eye patch. Intermittent double vision usually settles without surgery. Constant, persistent double vision can be treated surgically to adjust the pull of the affected muscle(s). Cosmetic surgery can adjust the position of the eyelids or remove puffy bags under the eyes. However, except with decompression, it is important to wait until the eye condition is stable and the thyroid hormone levels are consistently normal before undergoing surgery.

People with bad eye problems can find this waiting time distressing. It may seem as if your doctor does not care – why isn't he doing something? It is usually because things are not stable yet. Discuss exactly what is going on with your eye surgeon and thyroid adviser. Some eye surgeons have a special interest in thyroid ophthalmopathy. The TED Association (thyroid eye disease group) can help provide support (see page 167).

Causes

As with the thyrotoxicosis itself, the eye problems seem to be due to the formation of antibodies to the tissues behind the eye and the eye muscles. There is debate as to exactly what happens, but the end result is the building-up of gel-like compounds behind the eye, with swelling of the muscles which move the eye. This causes the eye to bulge forwards and limits the movement of the muscles. Fluid accumulates in and around the eye. The process waxes and wanes on its own, making it difficult to evaluate different treatments.

Summary

- Minor eye changes, for example puffy eyelids, can occur because of thyroid overactivity or thyroid underactivity. These changes resolve with treatment of the thyroid problem.
- A separate, sometimes more serious, eye problem can occur in people with thyroid disease (Graves' disease) or on its own.
- In Graves' eye disease there may be lid lag, lid retraction and exophthalmos – eye protrusion. In more severe cases double vision or visual impairment may occur.
- In most cases, the eye problems settle without medical intervention. In a few people, additional treatment is needed.
- It is important to keep the thyroid hormone levels normal in someone with thyroid eye disease.

17
Goitres and Nodules

A goitre is simply a swollen or enlarged thyroid gland; as the thyroid enlarges, for whatever reason, the neck fills out. But the swollen thyroid can also expand downwards behind the breastbone or sternum – this is called a retrosternal goitre. Teenage girls, young women and pregnant women may develop a slight fullness of the thyroid. This is completely harmless and does not indicate a thyroid disorder.

Smooth Soft Goitre

This is the sort of goitre that accompanies Graves' thyrotoxicosis. It may simply be a suggestion of fullness in the neck or an obvious swelling on both sides of the trachea. It is a very 'busy' goitre – you may be able to feel the blood rushing through as a vibration under your fingers and your doctor may be able to hear the increased blood flow as a thyroid bruit (see page 83). If you look at the thyroid tissue under a microscope, the follicular cells may be taller than usual and there may be holes in the colloid because it is turning over so fast. There are a lot of blood vessels. A thyrotoxic goitre does not hurt and it is rarely big enough to cause problems because of pressure in the neck.

A Multinodular Goitre

This sort of goitre is lumpy and irregular, and some parts of it may be quite firm. Most multinodular goitres are probably caused by iodine deficiency and occur commonly in countries where iodine is lacking. They occasionally can be caused by eating or drinking substances which block thyroid hormone production and sometimes by excessive iodine intake (such as eating a lot of seaweed). Sometimes thyrotoxicosis occurs, often in someone with long-standing multinodular goitre (see page 97).

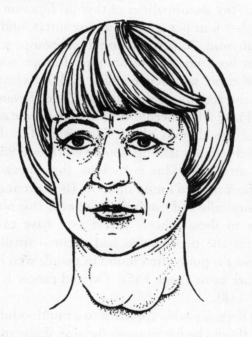

Multinodular goitre.

Multinodular goitres can grow large and may extend down behind the sternum. Occasionally the goitre presses on the trachea or gullet. Sometimes people feel as if they are wearing a tight collar. They may want to clear their throat or cough and limit breathing or swallowing; however, this is rare. What is more common is that once people have become aware of their goitre, they then start to feel discomfort in their neck, even though the goitre is not actually pressing on anything.

A recent European survey of the management of non-toxic multinoduiar goitre showed considerable variation in the ways in which doctors who were members of the European Thyroid Association would investigate and treat the condition. All would measure thyroid function using blood tests. Any abnormalities of thyroid function are then treated. Eighty four per cent would use ultrasound scans to image the thyroid, 76 percent would use isotope scans, and 69 per cent both imaging techniques. Isotope scans use a tiny dose of either radioactive iodine 123 or technetium 99 to look at the activity of the thyroid gland. Seventeen per cent would take a fine needle sample (fine needle aspiration – FNA) of the thyroid gland. However, if a dominant nodule which did not take up isotope was found 93 per cent would do an FNA. This is to look for cancer. Hidden thyroid cancer may be found in up to 16 per cent of goitres removed surgically and carefully examined. It is not known how many to these cancers would ever have caused any problems for the person who had them – small, hidden thyroid cancer is quite often found in people who have died from another cause (page 145). Thyroid cancer is rare (see pages 145–148).

So what is a reasonable approach to a multinodular goitre. Your neck should be felt to assess the size, shape and texture of the thyroid, whether it goes below the breastbone (sternum), and whether there are any enlarged lymph nodes. Everyone should have blood tests for thyroid function. A suppressed TSH means that there is very unlikely to be any malignant change in the thyroid. It seems sensible to do an ultrasound and take FNAs from any nodules that can be felt or are over 1 cm in size. It may be easier to do this under ultrasound control. Ultrasound may also show cysts which can be drained. FNA uses a fine needle (similar to the one used to take blood from your arm) to take a tiny sample of tissue from the thyroid. This is a quick, minor procedure. It stings and may cause bruising. Very rarely, bleeding may occur. The sample is then sent to the laboratory for examination under the microscope. Techniques similar to those used for FNA can be used to drain cysts. These often gradually refill.

If the patient is thyrotoxic, an isotope scan will show if there is a single overactive nodule, or whether there is more general over activity. Nodules which show as overactive on iodine 123 scanning are very unlikely to be cancerous.

If the goitre is large, unsightly, or causing compression symptoms, surgical removal of most of the thyroid is usually advised. If any cancerous or doubtful cells are seen on FNA, surgical removal of the thyroid is usual. With an overactive "toxic" multinodular goitre, the overactivity is controlled with anti-thyroid drugs and then surgery or radioiodine are used (see Chapter 13). Cancer is rare in toxic goitres but can occur. So dominant or larger nodules should still be sampled by FNA. If the nodules found in the thyroid cannot be felt, and are under 1 cm in size, then the goitre can be monitored annually by examination and ultrasound scanning. If you have pain in your neck see your doctor. Occasionally blood can leak into a cyst or nodule which is rarely harmful but may hurt.

Solitary thyroid nodules

Sometimes a part of the thyroid starts growing on its own. This forms a solitary thyroid nodule. Such nodules are usually harmless – less than 10 per cent are cancerous. Men, and those under 20 or over 60 years of age are more likely to have a cancerous noduie than other people. Previous irradiation of the neck, and a family history of thyroid cancer also predispose to thyroid cancer. Symptoms which should be investigated promptly are hoarseness, difficulty in swallowing or breathlessness. A nodule which has grown fast, or is over 5 cm in diameter, or is hard and irregular is more likely to be cancerous, as is one associated with enlarged lymph glands in the neck. However, some benign nodules become hardened by calcium. Sometimes what has formed is a cyst, not a nodule. This may swell fast as it fills with fluid, is usually harmless, and can be drained (see above).

A survey of members of the European Thyroid Association showed that doctors vary in their approach to solitary thyroid nodules. Nearly all would check thyroid function on a blood test. Ninety-nine per cent would take a FNA from the nodule, either straightaway in the clinic; or under ultrasound control (42 per cent). An ultrasound scan would be arranged by 80 per cent. Sixty six per cent would request an isotope scan to see if the nodule is overactive or not.

The FNA will usually show one of four results. Most FNAs show normal thyroid tissue. At least 10 per cent of FNAs will be reported as nondiagnostic – there was too little thyroid tissue for analysis, in which case the FNA must be repeated.

Occasionally, follicular or Hurthle cell abnormalities will be reported. Hurthle cells are rare and look pale under the microscope. Although most nodules with these cells are benign, about 10 to 20 per cent are malignant, although it can be hard to assess this sometimes. The American Thyroid Association suggests that follicular or Hurthle cell nodules should be imaged with a radioactive iodine 123 scan. If this shows overactivity the chance of malignancy is minimal and they can be treated with radioiodine (131) if the patient is thyrotoxic. If the follicular or Hurthle cell nodule is not overactive it can be removed surgically, although some people would try to shrink it with thyroxine treatment. This is becoming less popular because of the possibility of making the patient thyrotoxic and therefore risking the complications of thyrotoxicosis.

Less than 10 per cent of thyroid nodules are cancerous on

FNA. These should be removed surgically (see the section on thyroid cancer). In the survey of members of the European Thyroid Association, most doctors would opt for surgical treatment of any nodule with a high risk factors for malignancy (see page 169), regardless of FNA results.

Thyroid nodules are very common if you look hard enough. One study examined the thyroid glands of people who had died from any cause and found that one in two contained nodules. Thus half of us have thyroid nodules of which we are unaware and which do us no harm at all. If you have a thyroid nodule it is likely that it is harmless.

Thyroid Cancer

Everyone with a lump worries about cancer. Thyroid cancer is rarely found – it is diagnosed in about four people per 100,000 a year. However, post-mortem studies in which the thyroid glands of people who died from any cause were examined extremely carefully showed that as many as one in four people have tiny cancers hidden in their thyroid gland – usually the papillary variant (see page 146). These cancers have not caused any harm and would not have been found without very detailed microscopic examination. However, if thyroid cancer is found in someone it is always treated to be on the safe side.

Thyroid nodules are uncommon in children but one in two of those found in children aged under 14 years are cancerous. A new thyroid nodule in an elderly person should also be treated with suspicion. If you have a family history of thyroid cancer (a very rare situation) you should be followed by a specialist centre as these families may have multiple hormone problems (see page 154). Enlarged lymph glands in the neck of someone with a thyroid nodule may be associated with papillary cancer – but remember that we can all get enlarged lymph glands in the neck from time to time, with a sore throat or viral illness, for example.

Thyroid cancers are divided into papillary (about 75 per cent of thyroid cancers), follicular (about 10 per cent), anaplastic and medullary, depending on the sort of cells they contain. It can be very difficult to decide what sort of cancer it is, even for an expert – some seem to be mixed sorts.

Papillary thyroid cancers usually have a good prognosis. Good signs are being a women, tumours under 2 cms in diameter, and those without local or distant spread. Papillary tumours grow slowly. A surgeon will remove the lobe containing the tumour and the isthmus. Indeed, most thyroid surgeons would nowadays remove the whole thyroid, just preserving the parathyroid glands. A total thyroidectomy increases the risk of damage to parathyroid glands, and damage to other neck structures such as the recurrent laryngeal nerve. It is important that such operations are performed by a surgeon experienced in thyroid surgery. If there are any enlarged neck lymph nodes these will usually be removed too. Most people with evidence of spread of the cancer outside the thyroid would be given a large dose of radioiodine 131 to destroy any remaining thyroid tissue.

After surgery (with or without radioiodine) you will need lifelong thyroxine replacement at doses aiming to suppress TSH to remove any stimulus for growth of any residual thyroid tissue. The aim is to keep the TSH suppressed without overt thyrotoxicosis. Thus your blood thyroid hormone levels must be monitored regularly. You are likely to need calcium replacement too, with monitoring of blood calcium levels. Monitoring should be done by a doctor familiar with the management of patients with thyroid cancer. After surgery tests usually include measurement of blood thyroglobulin levels to check for the presence of residual, or increasing functioning thyroid tissue. Whole body radioiodine scans are performed to check for evidence of residual thyroid or distant spread. Before any radioiodine treatment or scan your thyroxine replacement will be changed to T3 treatment which is then stopped altogether for two weeks or until your TSH is over 30 mu/1 to allow optimal uptake of radioiodine. If you are a woman of childbearing age you must have a pregnancy test before radioiodine.

Follicular thyroid cancer is divided into invasive, and minimally invasive forms. Invasive follicular cancer is one which has spread beyond the capsule or membrane around the nodule. This is treated in a similar way to papillary cancer. Minimally invasive follicular cancer has not spread beyond the capsule and has an extremely good prognosis. Some endocrinologists would treat it in the same way as invasive cancer, others would remove the thyroid lobe only and either give suppressant thyroxine alone, or radioiodine ablation with subsequent radioiodine scans.

Medullary cell thyroid cancer is uncommon. About one in four patients with this will have a family history of thyroid cancer. If medullary thyroid cancer is found the whole family must see an endocrinologist specialising in this condition (which forms part of a rare problem called multiple endocrine neoplasia) for checks. In some families one in two first degree relatives will have the condition. There are now genetic tests for this. Medullary carcinoma of the thyroid can be associated with other rare hormone conditions such as phaeochromocytoma. This is an adrenaline-producing tumour which can cause blood pressure surges and collapse during operations if undetected, so checks must always be done. The test for phaeo-chromocytoma is a 24-hour urine collection to measure adrenaline byproducts.

Anaplastic thyroid cancer is the rarest form of thyroid cancer and most endocrinologists will only see one or two such patients in their whole career. It is important to have a tissue sample to be certain of the diagnosis. Surgery, external radiation and chemotherapy have been tried, but the cancer usually progresses rapidly. Much can be done to relieve pain, and other symptoms. It does not run in families.

Lymphoma occasionally occurs in the thyroid. Such patients should see a haematologist (blood specialist) or a haematological oncologist – blood doctor specialising in tumours.

Thyroid cancer in perspective

I have written about thyroid cancer as there is often not much information for patients who have this. However, it should be remembered that a diagnosis of thyroid cancer is rare. I am talking about approximately four people per 100,000 a year. Thus in our large district of a quarter of a million people, only about ten will develop thyroid cancer next year. If thyroid cancer is found, it can usually be treated very effectively. Seventy-five per cent of people with papillary or follicular cancer survive over 30 years. In most people the diagnosis of thyroid cancer has little impact on longevity. Indeed, it is said that most patients with thyroid cancer will live longer than their doctor!

Thyroiditis

In acute thyroiditis (inflammation of the thyroid) your thyroid may swell and become hot and tender, you may have a sore throat and tender lymph glands in your neck, and you may have transient thyrotoxicosis and, later, myxoedema. Your thyroid usually returns to normal, but occasionally it may remain swollen and firm, although no longer tender. This may be called de Quervain's thyroiditis.

There is also a form of thyroiditis in which the thyroid

becomes moderately swollen and very hard. Eventually you may become myxoedematous.

Summary

- A goitre is a thyroid swelling. If you notice that your thyroid is swollen, ask your doctor to check it.
- Girls, young women or pregnant women often have slightly swollen thyroid glands.
- A smooth, soft, symmetrical goitre is common in people with thyrotoxicosis.
- Multinodular goitres can become large and occasionally cause pressure effects.
- Solitary thyroid nodules can be cystic or solid. They need further investigation. The majority are harmless.
- Thyroid cancer is rare. It can usually be treated effectively with a good prognosis.
- Thyroid inflammation, thyroiditis, may cause painful thyroid swelling that settles.

18

Conditions Associated with Thyroid Disorders

Many thyroid disorders are due to autoimmune problems – antibodies which destroy thyroid cells, causing myxoedema; and antibodies which stimulate thyroid hormone production, causing thyrotoxicosis, for example. If you have one autoimmune condition, you are more likely to have others than someone without an autoimmune problem. This chapter looks at conditions which sometimes occur in association with thyroid disorder. It summarises their signs and symptoms so that you can recognise them early if they happen to you. However, it is important to remember that most people with thyroid disorder do not get other problems.

Diabetes

Diabetes is a state of chronically high blood glucose level. Its proper name is diabetes mellitus (so called because the urine tastes sweet, like honey) to distinguish it from diabetes insipidus (tasteless urine). Diabetes insipidus is a rare pituitary disorder which I will not discuss further. Diabetes mellitus can occur at any age. There are two forms. Insulin dependent diabetes mellitus (Type 1), which is an autoimmune disorder, tends to occur in people under 40 years of age. Type 2 diabetes mellitus tends to occur in the over 40s. Type 2 diabetes is not thought to be due to autoimmunity. Type 1 diabetes always requires insulin treatment; Type 2 diabetes can usually be treated with tablets or diet alone. Over one in 10 people with diabetes has abnormal thyroid function.

In Type 1 diabetes antibodies destroy the insulin-producing islet cells and stop insulin production by the pancreas (a gland in the upper abdomen). In Type 2 diabetes the pancreas does not make enough insulin at the right time and the body tissues cannot use the insulin properly. Both conditions can be inherited.

The symptoms of diabetes are frequent urination, passing large volumes of dilute urine, thirst, weight loss (despite normal appetite), tiredness, tingling in hands or feet, blurred vision and constipation. Injuries and spots may take a long time to heal and you are more prone to infections, which take longer to resolve. Rarely, the body chemistry may be so deranged that you become comatose.

Diabetes is suggested by the presence of glucose in your urine and the diagnosis is confirmed by a raised blood glucose level.

The treatment of diabetes starts with a diet which contains little sugar or fat and plenty of starchy, high fibre carbohydrate such as bread, potatoes, rice and so on. People with Type 2 diabetes may need tablets (e.g. glibenclarnide, gliclazide, metformin) to lower the blood glucose towards normal. People with Type 1 diabetes cannot survive without insulin injections. There are many different types of insulin on the market with insulin pens to make injections easier. Most people with diabetes monitor their own blood glucose using a strip read by a meter or by eye and a tiny drop of blood from a fingerprick. Treatment is usually lifelong.

Diabetes can lead to tissue damage over the years – problems with the eyes, kidneys and nerves (e.g. those supplying the feet), foot problems such as ulcers, circulatory problems and coronary heart disease. Much of the tissue damage can be prevented or reduced by good diabetes self- care.

Addison's Disease

This is a rare condition in which the adrenal glands found on top of the kidneys are attacked by antibodies (or damaged by infection or surgery, for example). They stop making steroid hormones and the blood cortisol levels fall. We need steroids to respond to emergencies such as infection as well as to keep our salt and water balance normal. Addison's disease occurs in fewer than one in 100,000 people.

The symptoms of Addison's disease are tiredness, weakness, loss of energy, dizziness or faintness on standing, loss of appetite, weight loss, increased skin pigmentation, nausea, vomiting, diarrhoea, muscle aches and, rarely, collapse. A doctor may also find that your blood pressure falls on standing, and you have a low blood sodium level and a raised potassium level.

If you are very ill, the diagnosis can be made on a single blood cortisol level – it is low when it should be very high. Otherwise a Synacthen test is performed, injecting synthetic adrenocorticotrophic hormone – usually made in the pituitary – to stimulate adrenal cortisol production. This should cause a rise in the blood cortisol levels but cannot do so if the adrenal glands are not working.

The treatment is steroid tablets such as hydrocortisone and fludrocortisone. These must be taken every day without fail and doubled if you are ill. Most people start to feel much better within days of starting treatment. Steroid replacement treatment is usually lifelong.

Pernicious Anaemia

Pernicious anaemia occurs in under 1 per cent of the population over 45 years old. It is found in about 10 per cent of people with myxoedema and 1 per cent of those with thyrotoxicosis. Pernicious anaemia is due to vitamin B12 deficiency. For most of us (unless we are vegans) there is plenty of vitamin B12 in the food we eat. The vitamin B12 is absorbed from the stomach with the help of a chemical called intrinsic factor which is made in the stomach by gastric parietal cells. Antibodies to intrinsic factor and gastric parietal cells stop absorption of B12. About a third of people with autoimmune myxoedema have a gastric parietal cell antibodies but only a few will become B12 deficient. Vitamin B12 is essential for the production of red blood cells and its lack causes anaemia. It may also cause nerve and brain malfunction.

The symptoms of pernicious anaemia include those of anaemia – tiredness, paleness, breathlessness, dizziness. You may also experience loss of appetite, loss of weight, indigestion, diarrhoea, numbness of the feet and lower legs, loss of drive, psychiatric symptoms and poor memory or confusion.

Your doctor may find you to be very pale, with loss of sensation in the legs and psychological problems, even dementia. You may have a fever.

A blood count showing low haemoglobin and large red blood cells strongly suggests the diagnosis, which is proved by measuring vitamin B12 levels. Other, more detailed tests may be done.

The treatment is vitamin B12 injections every few months. The response is often dramatic – both in disappearance of the anaemia and the relief of other symptoms. The treatment is lifelong.

There are other causes of vitamin B12 deficiency which may need additional treatment. People with pernicious anaemia do not make as much gastric acid as other people and are slightly more prone to stomach cancer than the rest of the population. Any indigestion should be investigated promptly.

Rheumatoid Arthritis

This is a form of arthritis with inflammation of the linings of the joints, but other tissues in the body can also become inflamed. Rheumatoid arthritis occurs in 0.3 per cent of the population and can affect people of all ages. Rheumatoid arthritis is much less common than osteoarthritis (the 'wear and tear' arthritis). It occurs slightly more commonly in people with autoimmune diseases than might be expected by chance. The cause of rheumatoid arthritis is not clear, although there is an inherited component. About 1 to 4 per cent of people with thyrotoxicosis have been found to have rheumatoid arthritis and about 3 per cent of those with myxoedema may have it. However, others have not found a link.

The symptoms of rheumatoid arthritis include pain, swelling, and stiffness (especially morning) of joints. The distant joints of the hands and feet are particularly affected, but the wrists, ankles, knees and neck are also affected. Other joints are less commonly involved. Other problems include skin nodules, eye changes, anaemia, blood vessel inflammation, lung and heart involvement, nerve damage and, rarely, liver and kidney disorders.

Rheumatoid arthritis is diagnosed by the characteristic pattern of joint symptoms and signs with appropriate X-ray changes, rheumatoid nodules in the skin and a positive rheumatoid factor blood test.

A variety of drugs are used to treat rheumatoid arthritis, including pain-killers such as paracetamol. Non-steroidal anti-inflammatory drugs such as aspirin or ibuprofen are also used. Anti-malarials, gold salts and immunosuppressive drugs are also used. Surgery may be indicated for joint deformities and sometimes joint replacement. Treatment has advanced substantially in recent years and can slow down the disease process.

Vitiligo

Vitiligo means patches of pale skin which do not tan. Indeed, they may become severely sunburned without careful protection from the sun. The cells which produce the brown pigment, melanin, do not work. People with vitiligo have a tendency to autoimmune problems. The white patches can cause embarrassment, especially in otherwise dark-skinned people. They can be covered with specialist makeup if you feel they are a problem. Vitiligo is not dangerous in any way apart from the risk of sunburn. It is definitely not infectious.

Multiple Endocrine Neoplasias (see page 147)

These are very rare conditions. In type 2a medullary cardnoma of the thyroid is linked with phaeochromocytoma (a condition in which excess adrenaline is produced) and parathyroid tumours. In type 2b medullary carcinoma of the thyroid is linked with phaeochromocytoma and abnormalities of the mucosa, tall, thin body shape and eye and bowel abnormalities.

Summary

- People with one autoimmune condition may have others.
- Diabetes, pernicious anaemia, Addison's disease, vitiligo and rheumatoid arthritis have all been found more commonly in people with thyroid disorders than in the general population.
- Although you are unlikely to have one of these conditions, awareness of the symptoms may allow faster recognition and earlier treatment if they do occur.

19

Looking After Yourself

If you have thyroid disease you can do a lot to help look after yourself. You can keep yourself generally fit and can monitor your own condition – why wait until the next visit to the clinic before discovering that your thyroid has become overactive again? Why wait to learn that an increase in thyroxine is indicated? That is what this book is for, to help you to help yourself.

Keeping Fit

To keep fit you need to eat and sleep well and exercise and relax regularly.

Your diet

The first thing to consider is your weight. Is it right for your height or are you too fat or too thin? If you are underweight because you have thyrotoxicosis, for example, you need to eat large amounts of healthy food to regain your proper weight. If you are overweight because you have myxoedema, some of it will be fluid, and will disappear quite quickly with thyroxine treatment, but some of it may be fat, especially if you were overweight to start with. So watch the total amount you eat until the situation has become clear.

The food that we eat includes carbohydrate (starchy or

sugary foods), protein (e.g. meat, fish), fats (e.g. butter, olive oil), fibre (e.g. in vegetables, pulses like peas, or wholemeal products), minerals and vitamins. We need to think about what we eat, and how much we eat. Most of what is on our plate should be high fibre, starchy carbohydrate, with plenty of vegetables, small helpings of protein-containing foods, and very little fat. If you want to put weight on have a big plate. If you want to lose weight have a little plate.

The sort of carbohydrates which are best are those which take a long time to digest, such as pulses and beans, wholemeal bread and pasta, brown rice, potatoes in their jackets. Try not to eat much sugary carbohydrate food like biscuits, sweets, candies and cakes, nor sugar itself.

The best sort of fat to eat is polyunsaturated fat or oils e.g. sunflower or monounsaturated oils like olive oil. Avoid animal fat like cream, meat fat, hard cheese and butter. Choose low-fat protein options like chicken, turkey, white fish or soya. It is especially important to have a low-fat diet if you have myxoedema.

If you have a poor appetite, make small attractive meals to tempt your palate. If you have a huge appetite, try not to snack on chocolate or sweet biscuits, but choose healthier options.

Eat five portions of fruit and vegetables each day, more if you are constipated because of myxoedema.

Alcohol

You can have alcoholic drinks, but in moderation. This means fewer than 21 units a week for men and fewer than 14 units a week for women. A unit of alcohol is half a pint of beer or lager, a glass of wine, or a single measure of spirits.

Smoking

This is extremely dangerous for your health, whether you

have thyroid disorder or not. Smoking may worsen some thyroid problems, such as eye disease. One in two people who smoke will die from a smoking-related illness. However, if you have myxoedema you already have a high cholesterol level, which increases the risk of atherosclerosis (page 67). Smoking carries its own major risk of fat deposition in arteries, and therefore greatly increases the risk of heart or artery disease in people with myxoedema.

Stop smoking straightaway.

Weight

Nowadays, doctors calculate your weight according to your height using a formula called body mass index. This should be between 18 and 25 kilograms (kg) per metre (m) squared. Thus someone who weighs 72 kg at a height of 1.8 m has a body mass index of $72/(1.8 \times 1.8) = 22.2$. Many of us still think in stones and feet and inches. One kg = 2.2 pounds. One stone = 6.4 kg. One inch = 2.54 cm. One foot = 30.5 cm. A simple table is shown below.

Table 19.1 Examples of height and weight which give a body mass index from 18 to 25 kg/m^2 (healthy weight range).

Height		Weight	
1.52 m	(5 ft 0 ins)	42–46 kg	(6 st 8 lbs–7st 3 lbs)
1.67 m	(5 ft 6 ins)	50–70 kg	(7 st 12 lbs–10 st 13 lbs)
1.83 m	(6 ft 0 ins)	60–84 kg	(9 st 7 lbs–13 st 2 lbs)

Exercise

It is always important to keep your body, heart and lungs in trim. However, one of the problems of thyroid disorder is that you may not feel strong enough to exercise. Your muscles can be weakened by both overactivity and underactivity of the thyroid. They may ache, as may your joints. If the thyroid problem has affected your heart you may become breathless with exercise.

Whatever exercise programme you decide upon, it must be tailored to your individual fitness level, heart state and needs; it should be graded to prevent any undue strain on your body. This means that you must discuss your exercise plans with your doctor before you start.

Stress and relaxation

We live in a stressful world and many of us are exposed (or perhaps, more honestly, expose ourselves) to relentless pressures. Coping with stress as well as illness can be exhausting. It may delay your recovery.

Thyroid disorders may make you feel very unwell and until the treatment has started to take effect you should reduce the external demands on you. It may be best to stop work for a few weeks. Women should enlist their families' help with the household chores; this is particularly important if your thyroid trouble has occurred with the arrival of a new baby. Try to relax, whether your thyroid is overactive or underactive.

People with myxoedema usually have no problem relaxing – their problem is getting themselves going. In contrast, people with thyrotoxicosis often find it very difficult to relax – the thyroid hormone excess pushes them on relentlessly. As your thyroid overactivity comes under control, set aside a time each day to relax completely; try to sit comfortably, or lie down for the whole of your set time.

Decision-Making

Because thyroid hormones affect the working of the whole body, they can affect the way you plan and decide things. Your memory may be poorer than usual. If your thyroid is overactive you may find it hard to concentrate on a single problem; if you are myxoedematous you may just fall asleep while you are thinking.

It is therefore important to realise that there may be a period of time – weeks or a month or so – when your mind is not as razor-sharp as you would wish. Things will improve rapidly as your treatment takes effect. However, while you are waiting to feel better, try to avoid decisions unless you cannot put them off. If you have to decide something right now, share the problem with someone you trust. Obviously some people experience more effects from thyroid hormone lack or excess than others – but be aware that you yourself may not be the best judge of your own decision-making capabilities while you are unwell.

Monitoring your Thyroid

It may help you and your doctor to keep a little diary of the progress of your thyroid condition. You may need treatment for ever if you have permanent myxoedema, or for many years if you have thyrotoxicosis. It can be difficult to recall what happened when, and which pills you took for how long. But if you have written notes of things you can measure, like your weight or pulse, as well as how you feel, you can see if your thyroid function is speeding up, slowing down or steady. But do not overdo this – keep things in perspective; a brief note of any events or changes and a few regular observations are all that is needed.

Weight

At the beginning measure your height and work out what weight range is acceptable for you (see page 158).

If you do not already have some bathroom scales, buy some and use them according to instructions – they should be on a flat even surface for best results. Make sure you know how to zero them. Get into the habit of weighing yourself regularly, say once a week or once a fortnight. It is best to choose the same time of day, with nothing on.

Pulse rate

The easiest pulse to measure is the one at your wrist – the radial pulse.

Hold your hand, palm up, and follow your thumb down to its base at the wrist crease. Two or three centimetres (about an inch) beyond this, in a groove between the tendons and the side of the wrist, is the radial pulse. Feel it lightly with the fingers of the other hand – it may take a few seconds to become obvious. Using a watch with a second hand, count the number of beats for a minute. Count your pulse when you are resting in bed at night or on waking. The normal range varies depending on how fit you are, how rested you are and how anxious you are. In bed it should be between about 60 to 80 beats per minute.

You should be particularly interested in the trend of your heart rate. Is it getting faster or slower over succeeding months? Is it much the same? Count your pulse on the day when you weigh yourself and write it down. Note down whether the rhythm is regular (the beats feel like * * * * * * *) or irregular (the beats may feel like this ** * * *** * ** *).

Neck circumference

Only measure this if you have a goitre. Use a tape measure and gently put it round your neck where it is widest, i.e. at the bulge of the goitre. Make sure hair, necklaces, etc. are out of the way. Note down the measurement about once a month.

General observations

- Has your face changed at all? Is it fatter or thinner? Is it pale?
- Are your eyelids swollen? Do you have lid retraction (page 135)? Look straight ahead and keep your eyelids relaxed to check. Are your eyes bulging? Are they bloodshot? Do you have double vision?
- Is your skin dry and cold, or hot and sweaty? Have you got patches of swollen or lumpy skin? Have you got a rash?
- Is your hair coarse, fine, difficult to handle, coming out?
- Are your nails brittle, a funny shape, hard to keep clean?
- Are your hands puffy or shaky?
- Are your ankles or feet puffy?
- Are your muscles weak? Can you stand up from squatting without using your hands?

Symptoms

One of the problems about encouraging people to take an interest in their bodies is that they suddenly have symptoms everywhere. Medical students and doctors are always misdiagnosing serious diseases in themselves – it is an occupational hazard. Pulled chest muscles turn into heart attacks; a headache becomes a brain tumour. I do not want to encourage you to worry over every minor symptom, but it is useful to note some of the more specific symptoms which might indicate that the thyroid gland is becoming overactive or underactive, or that it has returned to normal.

- *Temperature preference* Do you feel the heat or the cold more than other people around you?
- *Tiredness* Do you go to bed at the same time as everyone else, or earlier or later? Do you have to go to bed during the daytime (nightshift workers excluded)?
- *Chest pain* If you have any pain in your chest, contact your

doctor straightaway. But do not be frightened; remember that most chest pains are not heart attacks.

- *Palpitations* If you are unduly aware of your heart's action, feel your pulse and note the rate and rhythm.
- *Appetite* Do you find it hard to clear one plateful or do you ask for second helpings?
- *Bowels* Approximately how often do you open your bowels each day or how many days are there between each motion? There is a wide range of normal bowel habits – you do not have to go every day. The main thing to notice is if there is any change from your usual bowel habit.
- *Periods* Premenopausal women should note down the date on which each period starts and finishes.

If you have any other symptoms note them down to discuss with your doctor see the tables on pages 14 and 70. You do not have to have any symptoms – the aim is for you to be feeling fine.

Check-ups

The frequency of your medical checks will be organised by your doctor. In the United Kingdom you will be under the care of a general practitioner, who may investigate and treat you himself or who may refer you to an endocrinologist – a hormone specialist in a hospital. The specialist may continue to see you in his or her clinic, or may return you to your general practitioner.

Ask your doctor for the most recent results of your thyroid hormone tests and other investigations, and write them in your own record. Initially you may be seen at four to eight week intervals. Eventually you will be seen at longer intervals, perhaps annually. Long term, I personally feel that anyone who is receiving treatment for myxoedema or who has ever had thyrotoxicosis should see his or her doctor annually and have a blood test for thyroid hormone levels.

In most cases the general practitioner is happy to provide this follow up. If you are keeping an eye on yourself in between, you can ask for an early appointment at the first signs that your thyroid is misbehaving.

Summary

- You can do a lot to keep yourself healthy.
- Eat a low-fat diet and watch your weight
- Relax and avoid stress and important decisions until you are well enough to deal with them.
- Exercise regularly according to your doctor's advice.
- Keep an eye on your condition. Note dates, test results and treatments.
- Note any symptoms, but do not frighten yourself by imagining things. If you are not sure whether you can feel something or not, it is probably not there.
- Attend your medical check-ups and ask your doctor about anything you do not understand.
- Look after yourself.

Diabetes and Endocrine Unit
The Hillingdon Hospital

Your Thyroid

The thyroid is a gland in your neck which
makes two hormones – thyroxine (T4) and
tri-iodo thyronine (T3).

T3 and T4 production are controlled by the
pituitary gland in the head which makes
thyroid stimulating hormone (TSH).

If your thyroid is overactive your T4 and T3
will be high and your TSH will be low.
You may feel hot, sweaty, wound up, shaky;
have palpitations (a fast heart rate) and lose
weight.

If your thyroid is underactive your T4 and T3
will be low and your TSH will be high.
You may feel cool, slow, tired, constipated;
have dry skin and gain weight.

If the pituitary gland is not working T4, T3 and
TSH are low.

Thyroid Card

Name   No.

Allergies

Thyroid problem

Consultant: Dr. Hillson

DATE	WEIGHT	PULSE	FREE T4 (9–24)	FREE T3 (5.4–9.3)	TSH (0.3–5.0)	TREATMENT (INCLUDING ^{131}/SURGERY)

Contacts

American Thyroid Association
www.Thyroid.org

British Thyroid Foundation (BTF)
P.O. Box 97
Clifford
Wetherby
West Yorkshire LS23 6XD
Telephone 0870 770 7933
www.btf-thyroid.org

European Federation of Endocrine Societies
www.euro-endo.org

Pituitary Foundation
P.O. Box 1944
Bristol BS99 2UB
Telephone/Fax 0870 774 3355
www.Pituitary.org.uk

Society for endocrinology
17/18 The Courtyard
Woodlands
Bradley Stoke
Bristol BS32 4NQ
Telephone 01454 642200
Fax 01454 642222
www.endocrinology.org

This professional organisation provides links with various patient support groups for hormone problems.

Thyroid Eye Disease Association (TED)
Solstice
Sea Road
Winchelsea Beach
East Sussex TN36 4LH
Telephone 01797 222338
E-mail tedassn@eclipse.co.uk
www.thyroid-fed.org/members/TED.html

Thyroid Federation International
www.thyroid-fed.org

This federation has links with thyroid organisations worldwide. Full details can be found on their website.

These organisations and websites provide information about thyroid problems and other hormone disorders. The accuracy of this information has not been checked, and Dr Hillson does not endorse or take responsibility for information from these organisations.

References and
Further Reading

Tunbridge, W. M. G. *et al.* (1977) The spectrum of thyroid disease in a community. The Whickham survey, Clinical Endocrinology, 7, 481–93.

Allahabadia, A., Daykin, J., Holder, R. *et al.* (2000) Age and gender predict the outcome of treatment for Graves' Hyperthyroidism. Journal of Clinical Endocrinology and Metabolism, 85,1038–42

Allahabadia, A., Daykin, J. Sheppard, M. *et al.* (2001) Radioiodine treatment of hyperthyroidism – prognostic factors for outcome. Journal of Clinical Endocrinology and Metabolism, 86, 3611–7.

Franklyn, J.A., Maisonneuve, P., Sheppard, M. *et al.* (1999) Cancer incidence and mortality after radioiodine treatment for hyperthyroidism: a population-based cohort study. The Lancet. 353, 2111–5.

Franklyn, J.A. (1999). Thyroid disease and its treatment: short- and long-term consequences. Journal of Royal College of Physicians of London 33, 564-7.

Ron, E., Doody, M., Becker, D. *et al.* (1998). Cancer

mortality following treatment for adult hyperthyroidism. Journal of American Medical Association, 280, 347–55.

Royal College of Physicians (RCP) Guidelines. "The use of radioiodine in the management of thyrotoxicosis" November 1995.

Vanderpump, M.P.J. *et al.* (1996) on behalf of a working group of the Research Unit of the RCP London, the Endocrinoiogy and Diabetes Committees of the RCP London, and the Society for Endocrinology. "Consensus statement for good practice and audit measures in the management of hypothyroidism and hyperthyroidism." British Medical Journal, 313, 539–44.

Franklyn, J. (1999) Thyroid disease and its treatment: short- and long-term consequences. Journal of Royal College of Physicians of London 33, 564–7.

Girling, J. (2000). Thyroid disease in pregnancy. Hospital Medicine, 61, 835–40.

Lazarus, J. and Kokandi, A. (2000). Thyroid disease in pregnancy: a decade of change. Clinical Endocrinology. 53, 265–78.

Bennedbaek, F.N., Perrild, H. *et al.* (1999). Diagnosis and treatment of solitary thyroid nodule. Results of a European survey. Clinical Endocrinology, 50, 357–63.

Bonnema, S.J., Bennedbaek, F.N. *et al.* (2000) Management of the non-toxic multinodular goitre: a European questionnaire study. Clinical Endocrinology, 53, 5–12.

Kumar, H., Daykin, R. *et al.* (2001) An audit of management of differentiated thyroid cancer in specialist and non-specialist clinic settings. Clinical Endocrinology, 54, 719–23.

Lim, A.K.P, Daykin, R. *et al.* (1998) Measurement of serum TSH in the investigation of patients presenting with thyroid enlargement. Quarterly Journal of Medicine, 91, 687–9.

Miller, F.R., and Netterville, J.L. (1999). Surgicai management of thyroid and parathyroid disorders. Medical Clinics of North America. 83, 247–59.

Singer, P.A., Cooper, D.S. *et al.* (1996) Treatment guidelines for patients with thyroid nodules and well-differentiated thyroid cancer. Archives of Internal Medicine, 156, 2165–72.

Glossary

Medical words are defined within the context of this book. Some words may have other meanings in other contexts.

Addison's disease Condition due to failure of adrenal gland.

adrenal gland Gland found above the kidney which makes adrenaline and steroid hormones.

adrenaline (USA **epinephrine**) Flight, fright and fight hormone produced by the adrenal gland under stress.

allergy Abnormal sensitivity of the body to substances which are usually harmless. An allergic reaction usually produces unwanted symptoms.

anaemia (USA **anemia**) Lack of red blood cells.

angina Chest pain caused by insufficient blood supply to heart muscle (a form of ischaemic heart disease). Also known as angina pectoris.

ankle oedema (USA **edema**) Excess fluid in ankles, causing swelling.

antibody Chemical made by lymphocytes in response to an antigen.

antigen Chemical which triggers the body's defence mechanism and stimulates production of an antibody.

antimicrosomal antibody Antibody to tiny particles called microsomes in thyroid cells.

artery Vessel which carries blood from the heart to other parts of the body.

atherosclerosis Hardening and furring-up of the arteries.

atrial fibrillation Irregular quivering of the atria causing an irregular heartbeat.

atrium Upper chamber of the heart where the blood returning from the body collects. Plural atria.

autoimmunity Condition in which chemicals normally found in the body act as antigens and stimulate antibody formation.

beta-blocker Drug which reduces high blood pressure, steadies the heart and prevents angina. All the names of beta-blockers end in -olol, e.g. atenolol.

blood pressure BP. Pressure at which blood circulates in the arteries.

bloodstream Blood flowing around the body contained within the blood vessels.

bradycardia Slow heartbeat, usually less than 60 beats per minute.

bruit Abnormal noise heard through stethoscope, usually due to turbulent flow in blood vessel.

calcium Electrolyte found in blood. Needed for bone strength, muscle function and other body functions.

carbimazole Drug used to reduce thyroid hormone production in thyrotoxicosis.

carbohydrate CHO. Sugary or starchy food that is digested in the gut to produce simple sugars like glucose. Carbohydrate foods include candy or sweets, cakes, biscuits, soda pop, bread, rice, pasta, oats, beans, lentils.

cardiac To do with the heart.

cardiac failure Reduced functioning of the heart causing shortness of breath or ankle swelling.

cardiomyopathy Disease of the heart muscle.

carpal tunnel syndrome Numbness in fingers caused by compression of the median nerve as it passes through the fibrous tunnel at the wrist (carpus).

carrier protein Protein circulating in the blood or other body fluids to which a hormone is linked during transport from the gland where it is made to the tissue(s) where it acts.

cells The tiny building blocks from which the human body is made. Cell constituents are contained within a membrane.

cerebellum Part of the brain responsible for balance and other coordinating functions.

chemosis Swelling of the conjunctiva.

cholesterol A fat which circulates in the blood and is obtained from fats in food.

cold intolerance Undue sensitivity to cold.

colloid Gel-like substance within the thyroid follicle where thyroid hormones are stored.

congenital Something you are born with.

conjunctiva The white of the eye and the inner eyelid.

connective tissue Inactive tissue which links other tissues.

constipation Infrequent and/or hard bowel motions.

coronary artery Artery that supplies the heart muscle.

coronary thrombosis Clot in an artery supplying heart muscle.

cretinism Mental retardation due to congenital thyroid hormone deficiency.

cyanosis Blue coloration, e.g. cyanosed lips. Usually indicates oxygen lack.

cyst Hollow fluid-filled swelling.

de Quervain's thyroiditis One type of inflammation of the thyroid gland.

Derbyshire neck Goitre due to iodine deficiency previously found in people living in Derbyshire.

diabetes mellitus Condition in which the blood glucose concentration is above normal, causing passage of large amounts (diabetes = a siphon) of sweet urine (mellitus = sweet, like honey).

diarrhoea (USA **diarrhea**) Frequent and/or loose bowel motions.

diastolic blood pressure Blood pressure between heartbeats.

diet What you eat.

dietitian Trained professional who promotes a healthy diet and recommends dietary treatments.

diplopia Double vision.

effusion An abnormal outpouring of fluid within a body cavity.

electrocardiogram ECG (USA EKG) Recording of the electrical activity of the heart muscle as it contracts and relaxes.

electrolytes Blood chemicals such as sodium and potassium.

endocrine To do with the ductless glands (glands which deliver their hormones directly into the bloodstream). The thyroid is a ductless gland.

endocrinologist Doctor specialising in hormone disorders.

epinephrine see **adrenaline**.

epiphora Watering eyes.

exophthalmometer Device for measuring exophthalmos.

exophthalmos Abnormal protrusion of eyes.

fat Greasy or oily substance. Fatty foods include butter, margarine, cheese, cooking oil, fried foods.

fibre (USA **fiber**) Roughage in food. Found in beans, lentils, peas, bran, wholemeal flour, potatoes, etc.

follicle Ball of cells within the thyroid where thyroid hormones are made. (Other meanings in other contexts.)

follicular cells Cells out of which thyroid follicle is made, and that produce thyroid hormones.

free T3 See **free tri-iodothyronine**.

free T4 See **free thyroxine**.

free thyroxine Thyroxine that is not bound to thyroxine-binding globulin in the bloodstream.

free tri-iodothyronine Tri-iodothyronine that is not bound to thyroxine-binding globulin in the bloodstream.

gastrointestinal To do with the stomach and intestines.

gland Structure in the body that secretes chemicals.

glucose A simple sugar obtained from carbohydrates in food. Glucose circulates in the bloodstream and provides energy.

goitre (USA **goiter**) Thyroid swelling.

granulocytes White blood cells responsible for engulfing bacteria.

Graves' disease Combination of thyrotoxicosis, exophthalmos and goitre described by Graves.

gynaecomastia Development of breast tissue in men.

Hashimoto's thyroiditis An autoimmune inflammation of the thyroid – the commonest cause of myxoedema.

heart Muscular organ that pumps blood around the body.

heart attack General non-specific term for myocardial infarction or coronary thrombosis.

hormone A chemical made in one part of the body and acting in another part of the body.

Human chorionic gonadotrophin (hCG) Hormone produced during pregnancy.

hydrocele Fluid in the scrotum causing swelling.

hyper- High, above normal.

hyperemesis gravidarum Excessive vomiting in pregnancy.

hypertension High blood pressure.

hyperthyroidism Thyroid overactivity. High thyroid hormone concentrations.

hypo- Low, below normal.

hypoglycaemia Low blood glucose concentration.

hypotension Low blood pressure.

hypothalamus Part of the brain. It has several functions, one being production of thyrotrophin.

hypothermia Low body temperature.

hypothyroidism Thyroid underactivity. Low thyroid hormone concentrations.

impotence Difficulty in obtaining or maintaining a penile erection.

incoordination Lack of coordination.

infarction Condition in which a body tissue dies from lack of blood supply – irreversible.

iodine Chemical required for thyroid hormone manufacture.

iodine 131 or I^{131} Radioactive iodine used to treat thyrotoxicosis.

iris Coloured part of eye forming the ring which contracts or expands around the central pupil.

ischaemia Condition in which a body tissue has insufficient blood supply – reversible.

ischaemic heart disease An illness in which the blood supply to the heart muscle is insufficient.

isthmus Narrow neck of tissue connecting the left and right lobes of the thyroid.

jaundice Yellow coloration due to bile pigments.

Jod-Basedow phenomenon Hyperthyroidism induced by iodine in someone who was previously iodine-deficient

kilocalories Cals or kcals. A measure of energy, for example in food or used up in exercise.

kilojoules Another measure of energy. One kilocalorie = 4.2 kilojoules.

larynx Voice box.

left ventricle Chamber of the heart which pumps oxygenated blood into the aorta.

left ventricular failure Reduced functioning of the left pumping chamber of the heart causing fluid to build up in the lungs and shortness of breath.

leuconychia White nails.

leucotrichia White hair.

libido Sexual urge.

lid lag Slow descent of upper eyelid and downward gaze in someone with thyroid eye disease.

lid retraction Apparent drawing back of upper eyelid to show white of eye above iris in someone with thyroid eye disease.

lipid General name for fats found in the body.

liver Large organ in upper right abdomen that acts as energy store, chemical factory and detoxifying unit, and that produces bile.

lobe Part of thyroid.

Lugol's iodine solution Iodine preparation used in the treatment of thyrotoxicosis.

lymphocyte White blood cell that produces antibodies in response to an antigen.

malaise Feeling vaguely unwell or uncomfortable.

median nerve Nerve that supplies part of the hand.

metabolism The chemical processing of substances in the body.

microgram (=μ) One-millionth of a gram; one-thousandth of a milligram. Measure of weight.

milligram (mg) One-thousandth of a gram. Measure of weight.

millimol per litre (mmol/l) Measure of concentration of substances in the blood.

mitochondria Tiny structures in which many chemical reactions occur. They are found inside cells.

multinodular goitre Thyroid swelling with lots of lumps in it.

muscle wasting Loss of muscle bulk.

myocardial infarction Death of heart muscle caused by lack of blood supply.

myocardium Heart muscle.

myopathy Muscle disorder.

myxoedema (USA myxedema) Thyroid underactivity or hypothyroidism in which there is swelling which does not indent with finger pressure. Term used in this book for all forms of thyroid underactivity.

nerve Cable carrying signals to or from the brain and spinal cord.

neuroelectrophysiology Study of the way nerves work.

neuropathy Abnormality of the nerves.

nodule Single lump.

nutritionist Trained professional who studies diets. Nutritionists may be dietitians, and vice versa.

obese Overweight, fat.
obesity Condition of being overweight or fat.
oedema (USA **edema**) Swelling.
onycholysis Condition in which fingernails separate from the nail bed and break easily.
ophthalmic To do with the eye.
ophthalmic Graves' disease Eye protrusion without abnormal thyroid function.
ophthalmologist Doctor specialising in eye disorders.
ophthalmoplegia Paralysis of eye muscle. Usually causes double vision.
ophthalmoscope Magnifying torch with which the doctor looks into your eyes.
oral Taken by mouth.
osteoporosis Thinning of the bones.

palpitations Awareness of irregular or abnormally fast heartbeat.
paraesthesiae Pins and needles or tingling.
partial thyroidectomy Partial surgical removal of the thyroid gland.
-pathy Disease or abnormality, e.g. neuropathy, retinopathy.
Pendred's syndrome Rare inherited disorder with myxoedema, deafness and white hair.
pericardial effusion Fluid within the pericardium.
pericardium Membranous bag within which the heart beats.
pernicious anaemia Anaemia due to vitamin B12 deficiency.
phlebotomist Person who takes blood samples.
picomol per litre (pmol/l) A micromicromol or a thousand- millionth of a millimol. Unit of concentration of substances in the blood.
pituitary Gland in head that controls the function of most other endocrine glands.
pituitary stalk Thin stem of tissue connecting the pituitary gland to the hypothalamus.
plasma Clear fluid in which the red blood cells are suspended. It is separated off by centrifuging unclotted blood.
platelets Particles found in the bloodstream which are essential for blood clotting.
Plummer's nails Onycholysis.

polydipsia Drinking large volumes of fluid.

polyunsaturated fats Fats containing vegetable oils such as sunflower seed oil.

polyuria Passing large volumes of urine frequently.

postural hypotension Fall in blood pressure on standing.

potassium Essential blood chemical.

premyxoedema State that precedes myxoedema – TSH is raised and thyroid antibodies are present, but thyroid hormone levels are normal.

pretibial myxoedema Thickening or swelling of the skin, usually over the lower leg, in people with thyroid hormone abnormalities.

prolactin Milk-producing hormone made in the pituitary.

propranolol Beta-blocker drug used to relieve the symptoms of thyrotoxicosis.

propylthiouracil Drug that reduces the production of thyroid hormones. Used in the treatment of thyrotoxicosis.

protein Dietary constituent required for body growth and repair. Found in meat and cheese, for example.

proximal myopathy Myopathy or muscle disorder of the limb muscles closest to the trunk.

radioactive iodine Form of iodine that is radioactive. Used to treat thyrotoxicosis.

radioiodine Radioactive iodine.

receptor Place on the cell wall with which a chemical or hormone links.

rectal To do with the rectum.

rectum Back passage, which holds faeces just before they are passed.

recurrent laryngeal nerve Nerve that controls vocal cords in the larynx.

reflex Involuntary action.

renal To do with the kidney.

retina Light-sensitive tissue at the back of the eye.

retrosternal goitre Goitre that extends down behind the sternum or breastbone.

saturated fats Fats usually found in animal products such as those in dairy products, meat fat. Also in coconut and some other plants.

secrete Actively release a chemical, e.g. a hormone, into the circulation.

serum Clear fluid obtained when blood clots. On clotting some components of plasma are bound up in the blood clot Thus serum is different from plasma.

sign Something you can see, touch, smell or hear.

sodium Essential blood chemical.

sternum Breastbone.

steroid hormone A hormone produced by the adrenal gland.

subcutaneous The fatty tissues under the skin.

symptom Something a person experiences.

systolic blood pressure Pumping pressure.

T3 Abbreviation for tri-iodothyronine.

T4 Abbreviation for thyroxine.

tachycardia Unduly fast heart rate.

TBG Thyroxine-binding globulin.

tendon reflex Involuntary muscle contraction on tapping a tendon.

testosterone Male sex hormone.

thrombosis Clotting of blood.

thrombus A blood clot.

thyroglobulin Chemical to which T4 and T3 are bound during storage within the thyroid follicle in the thyroid gland.

thyroglobulin antibodies Antibodies targeted against thyroglobulin as an antigen.

thyroid Endocrine gland in neck.

thyroid acropachy Increased curvature of nails, found in association with thyrotoxicosis.

thyroid antibodies Antibodies targeted against antigens that form part of the thyroid gland.

thyroid bruit Noise heard through stethoscope due to blood flowing through engorged thyroid gland.

thyroid crisis State of collapse due to severe thyrotoxicosis.

thyroidectomy Surgical removal of thyroid gland.

thyroiditis Inflammation of the thyroid gland.

thyroid nodule Lump in thyroid. May be solid or fluid-filled.

thyroid-stimulating hormone Thyrotrophin or TSH. Made in the pituitary, it stimulates T3 and T4 production by the thyroid gland.

thyroid-stimulating immunoglobulin (TSI) Chemical that acts like TSH in stimulating thyroid hormone production.

thyroid storm Thyroid crisis.

thyrotoxicosis Thyroid overactivity or hyperthyroidism. Originally associated with severe illness, i.e. 'toxicosis', but now more generally used.

thyrotrophin Thyroid-stimulating hormone (TSH) made in the pituitary gland.

thyrotrophin-releasing hormone TRH. Made in the hypothalamus, it stimulates production of TSH by the pituitary.

thyroxine (T4) Hormone containing four iodine units made by the thyroid gland.

thyroxine-binding globulin Protein which carries thyroxine in the blood.

total T3 T3, or tri-iodothyronine, bound to its carrier protein.

total T4 T4, or thyroxine, bound to its carrier protein.

trachea Windpipe.

TRH Abbreviation for thyrotrophin-releasing hormone or TSH-releasing hormone.

triglyceride Form of fat that circulates in the bloodstream.

tri-iodothyronine (T3) Hormone containing three iodine units made by the thyroid gland and produced in some tissues from thyroxine. The active thyroid hormone.

TSH Abbreviation for thyroid-stimulating hormone.

TSI Thyroid-stimulating immunuglobulin.

ultrasound scan Scan of a part of the body using sound waves.

urea Blood chemical; waste substance excreted in urine.

ventricle Pumping chamber of heart.

visual acuity Sharpness of vision.

vitiligo Areas of white depigmented skin.

vocal cord Flap of muscle in larynx or voice box. Blowing air out past the variable closing and opening of the two vocal cords allows speech and singing.

xanthelasma Fatty plaque above or below eye.

xanthoma Fatty lump in skin or tendon.

Index